T0201231

Peripheral Artery Disease

Peripheral Artery Disease

Edited By

Emile R. Mohler, MD, MSVM, FACC, FAHA
University of Pennsylvania, Philadelphia, PA, USA

Michael R. Jaff, DO, FACP, FACC, FAHA, MSVM
Newton-Wellesley Hospital, Newton, MA, USA

Second Edition

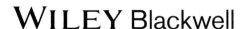

This second edition first published 2017 © 2017 by John Wiley & Sons Ltd.

Edition History

American College Of Physicians (1e, 2008)

The right of Emile R. Mohler and Michael R. Jaff to be identified as the author of the editorial material in this work has been asserted in accordance with law.

Registered Office(s)
John Wiley & Sons, Inc., 111 River Street, Hoboken, NJ 07030, USA

John Wiley & Sons Ltd, The Atrium, Southern Gate, Chichester, West Sussex, PO19 8SQ, UK

Editorial Office
9600 Garsington Road, Oxford, OX4 2DQ, UK
For details of our global editorial offices, customer services, and more information about Wiley products visit us at www.wiley.com.

Wiley also publishes its books in a variety of electronic formats and by print-on-demand. Some content that appears in standard print versions of this book may not be available in other formats.

Library of Congress Cataloging-in-Publication Data

Names: Mohler, Emile R., III, editor.
Title: Peripheral artery disease / edited by Emile R. Mohler, Michael R. Jaff.
Other titles: Peripheral arterial disease (Mohler)
Description: Second edition. | Hoboken, NJ, USA ; Chichester, West Sussex :
  John Wiley & Sons, Inc., 2017. | Preceded by: Peripheral arterial disease
  / edited by Emile R. Mohler III, Michael R. Jaff. Philadelphia : American
  College of Physicians, c2008. | Includes bibliographical references and
  index. |
Identifiers: LCCN 2017014491 (print) | LCCN 2017015849 (ebook) | ISBN
  9781118776070 (pdf) | ISBN 9781118776087 (epub) | ISBN 9781118776094
  (cloth)
Subjects: | MESH: Peripheral Arterial Disease--diagnosis | Peripheral
  Arterial Disease--therapy
Classification: LCC RC694 (ebook) | LCC RC694 (print) | NLM WG 550 | DDC
  616.1/31--dc23
LC record available at https://lccn.loc.gov/2017014491

Cover Design: Wiley
Cover Image: © Science Photo Library - SCIEPRO/Gettyimages

Set in 10/12pt Warnock by SPi Global, Chennai, India
Printed and bound in Malaysia by Vivar Printing Sdn Bhd

10 9 8 7 6 5 4 3 2 1

Contents

Contributors   *xi*
Preface   *xiii*

1   **Epidemiology of Peripheral Artery Disease**   *1*
Wobo Bekwelem and Alan T. Hirsch
Definitions   *1*
PAD Clinical Syndromes   *2*
Prevalence and Incidence   *3*
   Asymptomatic PAD   *8*
   Claudication   *10*
   Atypical Leg Pain   *12*
   Critical Limb Ischemia   *12*
   Acute Limb Ischemia   *13*
Risk Factors for Development of PAD   *13*
   Tobacco Use   *14*
   Diabetes Mellitus   *15*
   Dyslipidemia   *15*
   Hypertension   *16*
   Homocysteinemia   *16*
   C-Reactive Protein and Fibrinogen   *17*
   Obesity   *17*
   Other Risk Factors   *18*
Awareness of PAD in the Community   *20*
Progression, Natural History, and Outcomes of PAD   *20*
   Progression   *20*
   Natural History and Outcomes   *22*
Summary   *24*
References   *26*

2   **Office Evaluation of Peripheral Artery Disease – History and Physical Examination Strategies**   *37*
    Maen Nusair and Robert S. Dieter
    Introduction   *37*
    Identifying At-Risk Individuals   *37*
    Regional Symptom Analysis   *38*
        Neurologic Symptoms   *38*
        Thoracic Symptoms   *40*
        Abdominal Pain   *41*
        Extremity Pain   *42*
        Skin Manifestations   *44*
    Physical Examination   *46*
        General Appearance   *46*
        Head and Neck Examination   *46*
        Chest   *48*
        Abdominal Examination   *48*
        Lower Extremity Examination   *49*
        Palpating for Pulses   *50*
        Auscultation   *52*
    References   *53*

3   **Vascular Laboratory Evaluation of Peripheral Artery Disease**   *57*
    Thomas Rooke
    Introduction   *57*
        Anatomic   *57*
        Hemodynamic   *57*
        Functional   *58*
    Physiological Testing   *58*
        Background/History   *58*
            Physiological Invasive Testing   *58*
            Physiological Non-Invasive Testing   *58*
            Vascular Laboratory   *59*
        Doppler   *59*
            Motion Detection   *59*
            Waveform Analysis   *60*
        Plethysmography   *60*
            PVR Amplitude   *61*
            PVR Contour   *62*
        Ankle–Brachial Index (ABI) and Segmental Pressures   *63*
        Tissue Perfusion   *65*
        Transcutaneous Oximetry (TcPO$_2$)   *66*
    Duplex Scanning   *67*
        Background/History   *67*

Imaging (Anatomy)   *67*
Doppler (Hemodynamic)   *68*
Vascular Laboratory Accreditation   *69*
References   *69*

**4   Magnetic Resonance, Computed Tomographic, and Angiographic Imaging
of Peripheral Artery Disease**   *73*
Thomas Le, Masahiro Horikawa and John A. Kaufman
Introduction   *73*
Computed Tomography Angiography   *73*
  Basics   *73*
  Image Acquisition and Interpretation   *74*
    Protocol   *74*
  Advantages   *76*
  Pitfalls   *76*
    Calcification   *76*
    Artifacts   *76*
    Radiation Exposure   *76*
    Contrast-Induced Nephropathy   *76*
    Anaphylaxis   *77*
Magnetic Resonance Angiography   *77*
  Basics   *77*
  Image Acquisition and Interpretation   *77*
    Protocol   *77*
    Non-Contrast-Enhanced MRA   *77*
    Contrast-Enhanced MRA (CE-MRA)   *78*
    Post-Processing and Interpretation   *78*
  Advantages   *78*
  Pitfalls   *80*
    Time   *80*
    Nephrogenic Systemic Fibrosis   *80*
    Bolus Timing   *80*
    Artifacts   *80*
    Other Pitfalls   *80*
Conventional Angiography   *81*
  Basics   *81*
  Image Acquisition and Interpretation   *81*
    Pre-Procedure Patient Care   *81*
    Protocol   *81*
  Advantages   *82*
  Pitfalls   *82*
    Contrast-Induced Nephropathy and Anaphylaxis   *82*
    Artifacts   *84*

Other Disadvantages   *84*

Intravascular Ultrasonography   *84*

Basics   *84*

Advantages   *85*

Pitfalls   *85*

Results   *85*

Aortoiliac   *85*

CTA   *85*

MRA   *86*

Runoff   *86*

CTA   *86*

MRA   *86*

Pedal   *87*

CTA   *87*

MRA   *87*

Conclusion   *87*

References   *87*

5   **Non-atherosclerotic Peripheral Artery Disease**   *91*

Mitchell D. Weinberg and Ido Weinberg

Introduction – Presentation of Peripheral Artery Disease   *91*

When Should Non-atherosclerotic Causes of PAD Be Suspected?   *92*

Entities that Make up Non-atherosclerotic PAD   *94*

Popliteal Artery Entrapment Syndrome   *94*

External Iliac Artery Endofibrosis   *98*

Fibromuscular Dysplasia   *99*

Cystic Adventitial Disease   *100*

Vasculitis   *101*

Idiopathic Mid-aortic Syndrome   *102*

Arterial Manifestations of Pseudoxanthoma Elasticum   *102*

Chronic Exertional Compartment Syndrome   *103*

Musculoskeletal Pathology   *103*

Diagnostic Evaluation of Patients with Leg Pain with Exertion   *104*

Treatment Considerations   *105*

Conclusions   *105*

References   *105*

6   **Medical Therapy of Peripheral Artery Disease**   *111*

Lee Joseph and Esther S. H. Kim

Introduction   *111*

Atherosclerotic Risk Factor Management   *111*

Hypertension   *112*

Diabetes Mellitus   *113*

Hyperlipidemia   *114*
Tobacco Cessation   *114*
Antiplatelet Agents   *116*
Management of Claudication   *117*
Claudication Pharmacotherapy   *118*
Cilostazol   *118*
Exercise Therapy   *118*
Claudication Management Strategies: A Comparison   *119*
Lower Extremity Wound Care   *120*
Summary   *121*
References   *121*

7   **Endovascular Treatment of Peripheral Artery Disease**   *129*
Vikram Prasanna, Jay Giri and R. Kevin Rogers
Introduction   *129*
Clinical Background   *129*
Intermittent Claudication   *129*
Critical Limb Ischemia   *131*
Limb Prognosis/Overall Survival   *131*
Typical Anatomy in Patients with CLI   *131*
Patency Issues   *131*
Indications for Endovascular Therapy for CLI   *131*
Background for Endovascular Therapy   *132*
Anatomy   *132*
Technical Background   *136*
Preprocedural Imaging   *136*
Access   *138*
Anticoagulation   *139*
Antiplatelet Management   *141*
Radiation   *143*
Chronic Total Occlusions   *143*
Clinical Evidence for Peripheral Intervention   *145*
Aorto-Iliac Interventions   *145*
Angioplasty vs. Stent   *146*
Polytetrafluoroethylene (PTFE)-Covered versus Bare Metal Balloon-
Expandable Stents   *147*
Femoropopliteal Interventions   *147*
Angioplasty versus Stenting   *149*
Drug-Eluting Stents in Femoropopliteal Arteries   *149*
Drug-Coated Balloon (DCB) Therapy in Femoropopliteal
Disease   *150*
Covered Stents in Femoropopliteal Disease   *151*
Atherectomy   *152*

Specialty Balloons *153*
Tibioperoneal and Pedal Interventions *153*
Post-procedural Care *155*
Conclusion *155*
References *156*

8 Surgical Management of Peripheral Artery Disease *163*
Julia Glaser and Scott M. Damrauer
When to Refer Patients with Claudication *163*
When to Refer Patients with CLI *164*
Revascularization Options and Results *166*
Iliac Revascularizations *166*
Femoropopliteal Disease *169*
Tibioperoneal Disease *171*
Complications of Revascularization *173*
Preoperative Evaluation and Management *175*
Conclusion *175*
References *176*

Index *179*

Contributors

Wobo Bekwelem, MD MPH
Lillehei Heart Institute and
Cardiovascular Division
University of Minnesota Medical
School
Minneapolis
MN, USA

Scott M. Damrauer, MD
Hospital of the University of
Pennsylvania; and Corporal Michael
Crescent VA Medical Center
Philadelphia
PA, USA

Robert S. Dieter, MD RVT
Associate Professor of Medicine
Loyola University Medical Center
Maywood
IL, USA

Jay Giri, MD
Interventional Cardiology &
Vascular Medicine
Cardiovascular Medicine Division
University of Pennsylvania
PA, USA

Julia Glaser, MD
Hospital of the University of
Pennsylvania
Philadelphia
PA, USA

Alan T. Hirsch, MD
Director, Vascular Medicine, Quality
Outcomes, and Population Health
Professor of Medicine, Epidemiology
and Community Health
Lillehei Heart Institute and
Cardiovascular Division
University of Minnesota Medical
School
Minneapolis
MN, USA

Masahiro Horikawa, MD
Instructor, Dotter Interventional
Institute/Oregon Health & Science
University
Portland
OR, USA

Lee Joseph, MD MS
Division of Cardiovascular Diseases
Department of Internal Medicine
University of Iowa
Iowa City
IA, USA

Esther S.H. Kim, MD MPH
Cardiovascular Division
Vanderbilt University
Medical Center
Nashville
TN, USA

John A. Kaufman, MD MS
Frederick S. Keller Professor of
Interventional Radiology
Director of the Institute, Dotter
Interventional Institute/Oregon
Health & Science University
Portland
OR, USA

Thomas Le, MD MS
Assistant Professor, Department of
Radiological Sciences
David Geffen School of Medicine
at UCLA Los Angeles; and Staff
Interventional Radiologist
Section of Vascular and
Interventional Radiology
Department of Radiology
Olive View-UCLA Medical Center
Sylmar
CA, USA

Maen Nusair, MD
PeaceHealth Southwest Heart and
Vascular Center
Vancouver
WA, USA

Vikram Prasanna, MD
Interventional Cardiology &
Vascular Medicine
Cardiovascular Medicine Division
University of Pennsylvania
Philadelphia
PA, USA

R. Kevin Rogers, MD MSc
Section of Vascular Medicine and
Intervention
Division of Cardiology
University of Colorado
Aurora
CO, USA

Thomas Rooke, MD BS RVT
Krehbiel Professor of Vascular
Medicine
Mayo Clinic
Rochester
MN, USA

Ido Weinberg, MD FSVM
Vascular Medicine Section
Cardiology Division
Massachusetts General Hospital
Boston
MA, USA

Mitchell D. Weinberg, MD FACC
System Director of Peripheral
Vascular Intervention
Northwell Health System
Division of Cardiology; and
Assistant Professor, Hofstra
Northwell School of Medicine
Long Island
NY, USA

Preface

Peripheral artery disease (PAD) is unfortunately infrequently recognized. The treatment of PAD continues to evolve but is fundamentally focused on control of risk factors in order to prevent the associated risk of heart attack, stroke, and premature cardiovascular death as well as improvement in exercise performance and limb preservation. The pathophysiology of progressive atherosclerotic plaque in the extremities is thought to involve plaque hemorrhage and rupture, but few data support this presumption. Clinical research is needed to develop agents designed to halt progression of atherosclerotic disease in the peripheral arterial system. Despite these current limitations in understanding and treating PAD, new lipid modifying agents and new antiplatelet treatment of risk factors and strategies to improve pain-free walking distance have emerged, including the use of emerging endovascular strategies. In addition, with the rapid evolution of technology to improve arterial perfusion with minimally invasive catheter-based strategies, options for revascularization of patients with advanced symptoms and signs of PAD are improving.

The primary objective of *Peripheral Artery Disease* is to provide the reader with the most current information on diagnosis and treatment of PAD.

We hope that this reference provides an easy-to-use resource for the practicing clinician, ultimately resulting in better care for our patients. In addition, we would like to dedicate this entire book to Alan T. Hirsch, MD, who died suddenly and unexpectedly in April 2017. It minimizes his impact on the field and all vascular specialists to discuss his publications, presentations, and advocacy. Alan was a tireless voice for patients around the World who suffered from PAD. It was through his efforts that exercise and guidelines-based medical therapies have become primary in the management of these patients. We will forever miss his enthusiasm, humor, expertise and care, but most importantly, the World is a bit smaller with his passing.

1

Epidemiology of Peripheral Artery Disease

Wobo Bekwelem and Alan T. Hirsch

Lillehei Heart Institute and Cardiovascular Division, University of Minnesota Medical School, Minneapolis, MN, USA

This chapter describes the epidemiology of peripheral artery disease (PAD). The definitions used to describe PAD and PAD syndromes are discussed. The prevalence and incidence, risk factors, progression and outcomes of PAD are summarized. Finally, the low awareness of PAD in the community is highlighted.

Definitions

Peripheral artery disease is an all-encompassing term used to describe disorders of the structure (including stenosis and aneurysms) and function of all non-coronary arteries [1]. Peripheral artery disorders include atherosclerosis, plaque rupture, abnormal vascular reactivity, vasospasm, inflammation, arterial wall dysplasia, and thrombus formation leading to occlusion. In the past, a range of other terms have been used, including peripheral vascular disease (PVD), peripheral artery occlusive disease (PAOD), lower extremity arterial disease (LEAD), and arteriosclerosis obliterans. The term "PVD" is not synonymous as it is less specific, potentially signify venous, arterial or lymphatic disease. PAD is preferred as it communicates the accurate anatomic disease site, is accepted in all current practice guidelines, and better communicates the disease site to patients and other health care professionals.

Lower extremity atherosclerotic PAD is a marker of systemic atherosclerosis which begins in childhood [2] as deposits of cholesterol and cholesterol esters called "fatty streaks" begin to line the intima of large and medium-sized arteries. At this stage, atherosclerosis is subclinical, but it can be quantified using arterial ultrasound imaging in other vascular beds (e.g., the extracranial carotid arteries) to measure carotid intima media thickness (cIMT). Various cohort studies have demonstrated a higher prevalence of cardiovascular disease and increased incidence of poor cardiovascular outcomes in individuals with increased cIMT. This relationship of early atherosclerosis defined by cIMT measurements has been established in the Atherosclerosis in Communities (ARIC) study [3], the Osaka Follow-Up Study for Carotid Atherosclerosis 2 [4], the Cardiovascular Health Study (CHS) [5], the Rotterdam Study [6], the Tromsø study [7], and the Second Manifestations of ARTerial disease (SMART) study [8]. Progression of these fatty streaks by increased lipid accumulation, followed by development of a fibromuscular cap, lead to formation of a fibrous plaque. Risk factor exposure (e.g., smoking, diabetes, hypertension, diabetes, low high-density lipoprotein [HDL]-cholesterol concentrations, elevated non-HDL-cholesterol concentrations and obesity), lead to further progression of these atherosclerotic lesions and increase the risk of clinically manifest PAD and other atherosclerotic diseases [9]. Clinical PAD is detected when at least one infra-diaphragmatic stenosis leads to a measurable decrease in pedal systolic pressure measurements, with or without clinically recognized limb ischemic symptoms.

In this chapter, the term "PAD" is used exclusively to refer to partial or complete atherosclerotic obstruction of one or more lower extremity peripheral arteries.

PAD Clinical Syndromes

There are five recognized clinical syndromes of PAD that are characterized by distinct presentations. These syndromes are useful both in describing the epidemiology of PAD and in clinical care. They include:

- asymptomatic PAD
- classic claudication
- atypical leg pain
- acute limb ischemia (ALI)
- critical limb ischemia (CLI).

Approximately one-half of individuals with PAD may be asymptomatic, defined by the absence of self-reported leg symptoms [10–14], and this has important implications in estimating the accurate PAD prevalence. PAD in these individuals is defined by a low ($\leq$0.9) ankle–brachial index (ABI). The diagnosis of PAD is discussed in detail in Chapter 2. Claudication, which is the hallmark symptom of PAD, occurs in 10–35% [10–13] of individuals with PAD, and refers to the discomfort, pain, ache or fatigue in limb muscles that reproducibly occurs with exercise (e.g., walking) and is consistently relieved by rest [15]. Atypical leg pain is defined in individuals with objective evidence of PAD and who experience any leg symptom that is not classic claudication [16–18]. Up to

30–50% of individuals with PAD present with atypical pain [13, 15, 16]. ALI is defined by the clinical symptoms that arise with a sudden decrease in limb perfusion and that threatens the viability of the limb. While ALI is presumed to be an immediate vascular emergency, "acute" has been variably defined as occurring within 2 weeks of the initial ischemic presentation. ALI is usually due to thrombosis or embolism [19] and is clinically recognized by the "six Ps": pain, paresthesia, pallor, pulselessness, poikilothermia, and paralysis. It is estimated that 0.1–1% of PAD patients may experience an episode of ALI [20, 21]. CLI manifests as chronic (>2 weeks) ischemic rest pain, non-healing ulcer or gangrene in 1–2% of PAD patients [22].

Prevalence and Incidence

There are an estimated 202 million people living with PAD globally, with almost 70% of them residing in low- and middle-income countries. Current data suggest that the global prevalence of PAD may be increasing, from 164 million individuals in the decade beginning in 2000–2010, representing an overall 23.5% rise in PAD prevalence (28.7% in low- to medium-income countries [LMICs] and 13.1% in high-income countries [HICs]) [23]. PAD affects most adult populations worldwide irrespective of socioeconomic or national developmental status [24, 25]. Fowkes *et al.* [23] recently collated the global prevalence of PAD using data from 34 studies (12 from LMICs and 22 from HICs). In women aged 45–89 years old, PAD prevalence ranged from 2.7% to 24.2% in HICs, and from 3.96% to 18.65% in LMICs. In men aged 45–89 years old, PAD prevalence ranged from 2.76% to 24.77% in HICs, and from 1.21% to 21.5% in LMICs.

Overall, PAD incidence and prevalence rates are similar in high- and low- to middle-income countries. PAD is as much a problem in HICs as it is in LMICs. Although the rates are similar, due to the greater population of people that live in LMICs compared with HICs, the number of individuals with PAD in LMICs exceed that in HICs (140.8 vs. 61.2 million people) (Figure 1.1). PAD is much more prevalent than common cardiovascular diseases, such as heart failure and atrial fibrillation [23, 26, 27] (Figure 1.2). Various studies have estimated the prevalence of PAD using the presence of claudication, identification of low ABI in asymptomatic individuals, or evidence of advanced forms of PAD (ALI or CLI). It is important to note that the prevalence of PAD in a given population depends on the characteristics of the population studied (i.e., age, ethnicity, socioeconomic status, and risk factors) and the method of diagnosis. In 2007, Allison *et al.* [28] summarized race- and ethnicity-specific estimates of PAD prevalence. They used data from seven community-based studies (the Cardiovascular Health Study, Honolulu Heart Program, Multiethnic Study of Atherosclerosis, US National Health and Nutrition Examination Survey, San

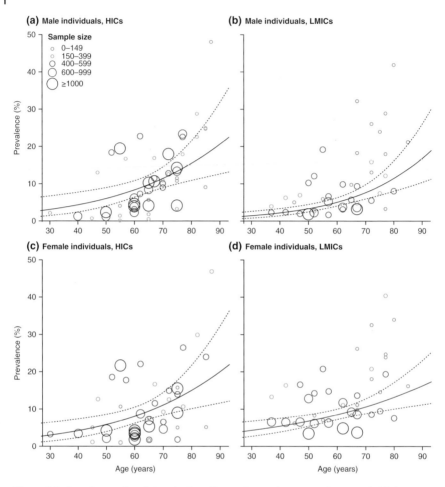

Figure 1.1 Prevalence of peripheral artery disease by age in men and women in high-income countries (HICs) and low- to middle-income countries (LMICs). *Source*: adapted from Fowkes *et al.* [23].

Diego PAD, San Diego Population Study and the Strong Heart Study). They found that with increasing age, the prevalence rates of PAD in men lay in the range 1.4–22.6% in non-Hispanic whites, 1.2–59% in blacks, 0.2–22.5% in Hispanics, 1.2–21.5% in Asians, and 2.6–28.7% in American Indians. PAD prevalence rates in women were in the range 1.9–18.2% in non-Hispanic whites, 3.0–65.1% in blacks, 0.3–18.2% in Hispanics, 0–18.2% in Asians, and 3.2–33.8% in American Indians. Eraso *et al.* [29] performed a multivariable age-, gender- and race/ethnicity-adjusted stratified analysis in this population, where the effect of each additional risk factor on the prevalence of PAD was

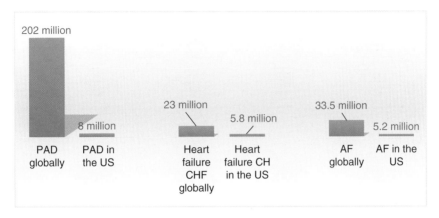

Figure 1.2 Comparison of the global and US prevalence of peripheral artery disease (PAD) and two other common cardiovascular diseases (congestive heart failure [CHF] and atrial fibrillation [AF]).

measured. Non-Hispanic blacks (odds ratio [OR] = 14.7, 95% CI: 2.1–104.1) and women (OR = 18.6, 95% CI: 7.1–48.7) had the highest odds of PAD as a result of this cumulative effect (Figure 1.3).

Due to the time and resources required to periodically retest study subjects for incident disease, fewer studies have evaluated the incidence of PAD. In 1970, Kannel *et al.* [30] assessed claudication incidence in the Framingham study. They reported the age-specific annual incidence of claudication for ages 30 to 44 years as 6/10 000 in men and 3/10 000 in women. The incidence increased among those aged 65–74 years to 61/10 000 in men and 54/10 000 in women. In 1988, the Edinburgh Artery Study used detection of claudication determined by the World Health Organization (WHO) questionnaire, the ABI, and a hyperemia test, among individuals aged 55–74 years, and reported an incidence of 15.5/1000 person-years. Hooi *et al.* [31] studied the incidence of asymptomatic PAD among 2327 Dutch subjects defined by an ABI < 0.9. After 7.2 years, the overall incidence rate for asymptomatic PAD was 9.9/1000 per-son-years. More recently, using data from CHS, Kennedy *et al.* [32] found that during 6 years of follow-up, incident PAD was detected in 9.5% of the cohort as defined by an ABI decrease of > 0.15 to a level of ≤ 0.90. Table 1.1 summarizes the available data on the age- and sex-specific incidences of PAD.

There have been significant methodological challenges relating to measuring the sex-based incidence of PAD. The male:female ratio of incident PAD is higher when measured based on claudication alone, with one study reporting a ratio as high as 1.97. However, in studies that have used an ABI definition of PAD, the incidence rates are lower for men (0.8) or similar between men and women (Table 1.1). Prevalent claudication is also more common in men than in women, with male:female ratio ranging from 1.2 to 2.38. However, when ABI

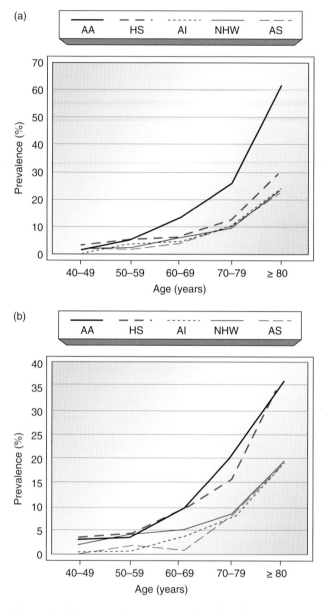

Figure 1.3 Ethnic-specific prevalence of peripheral arterial disease: (a) men; (b) women. AA, African American; AI, American Indian; AS, Asian American; HS, Hispanic; NHW, non-Hispanic white. *Source*: adapted with permission from Allison *et al.* [28].

Table 1.1 Age- and sex-specific incidence rates of peripheral artery disease measured by claudication and ankle–brachial index (ABI).

Study	Country	Mode of diagnosis	Age (years)	Annual incidence			
				Men	Women	Male:female	Overall
Ingolfsson et al. [33]	Iceland	Claudication	60	0.2%			
Bowlin et al. [34]	Israel	Claudication	60	1%			
Kannel and McGee [35]	US	Claudication	35–45	0.4/1000	0.2/1000		
			≥65	6/1000	6/1000		
			Overall	7.1/1000	3.6/1000	1.97	
Leng and Fowkes [36]	Scotland	Claudication	55–74				1.6%
Hooi et al. [31]	Netherlands	ABI < 0.95	40–54	1.7/1000	5.9/1000	0.3	
			55–64	1.5/1000	9.1/1000	0.2	
			≥65	17.8/1000	22.9/1000	0.8	
Nehler et al. [37]	US	ABI < 0.9**	Overall				2.35%

is used in PAD diagnosis, the overall prevalence is similar in both sexes, with a male:female ratio range of 0.8–1.2. The Multi-Ethnic Study of Atherosclerosis (MESA) [38] found that although the prevalence of PAD defined by a low ABI was similar in both sexes, borderline ABI (0.9–0.99) was much more common in women than in men (10.6% vs. 4.3%). Further, McDermott *et al.* [39] reported that atypical leg pain is more common in women. Fowkes *et al.* [23], in the global PAD report, found that male sex had an odds ratio of 1.43 for PAD in HICs and 0.5 for low-to-medium income countries. The global OR was 0.83. Although it is likely that overall PAD prevalence is similar in both sexes, men are more likely than women to have more classic claudication symptoms, while women are more likely to have borderline ABI, asymptomatic PAD and atypical symptoms [40].

Tables 1.1 and 1.2 summarize the available data on the worldwide prevalence and incidence of PAD based on the method of diagnosis.

Asymptomatic PAD

Asymptomatic PAD is defined as the presence of an ABI ≤ 0.9 without a clinically evident walking impairment or other leg symptoms. The ABI is performed

Table 1.2 Comparison of prevalence of claudication with prevalence of peripheral artery disease, with diagnosis based on ankle–brachial index (ABI).

Study	No. of patients	Age (years)	Prevalence of ABI abnormalities (%)	Prevalence of IC (%)
Reunanen *et al.* [15]	5738 men	30–59	–	2.1
	5224 women		–	1.8
Schroll and Munck [41]	360 men	60	16	5.8
	306 women		13	1.3
Newman *et al.* [42]	82 men	>60 (mean 72)	26.7	6.4
	105 women			
Fowkes *et al.* [12]	809 men	55–74	24.6	4.5
	783 women			
Newman *et al.* [42]	2214 men	65–85	14	2
	2870 women		11	
Zheng *et al.* [43]	6760 men	45–64	3	1
	8346 women		3.3	
Meijer *et al.* [44]	3052 men	70	16.9	2.2
	4663 women		20.5	1.2

IC, intermittent claudication.
Source: adapted from Cimminiello [45].

when the systolic blood pressures from both brachial arteries and that from both the dorsalis pedis and posterior tibial arteries are measured after the patient has been at rest in the supine position for 10 minutes using a continuous-wave Doppler device. It is computed as the ratio of each higher ankle to the higher of the two brachial systolic pressures. In healthy individuals, pulse wave reflection causes the ankle pressure to be 10–15 mmHg higher than the brachial arterial systolic pressure, and thus the normal ABI should be greater than 1.0. An ABI > 0.9 and < 1.4 is considered normal as these values are not associated with any detectable increase in cardiovascular ischemic risk (incident myocardial infarction [MI] or ischemic stroke). An ABI > 1.4 indicates non-compressible pedal vessels and an ABI ≤ 0.9 indicates hemodynamically significant arterial stenosis of the lower extremities [46]. The ABI will be addressed in more detail in Chapter 2, but we will briefly introduce the data showing validity of ABI in PAD diagnosis. The overall accuracy of the ABI to diagnose PAD has been well established. The comparative accuracy of an ABI threshold of 0.9 with angiography has been evaluated in various studies, notably by Fowkes *et al.* [47] and Lijmer *et al.* [48]. Fowkes *et al.* used an ABI threshold of 0.9 and showed that ABI has a sensitivity of 95% and a specificity of 100% compared with angiography to detect a ≥ 50% stenosis in peripheral arteries. Based on a receiver operating characteristic (ROC) analysis, Lijmer *et al.* demonstrated that an ABI threshold of 0.91 had a sensitivity of 79% and specificity of 96% to detect a 50% reduction in peripheral artery diameter. Multiple studies have also evaluated the inter- and intra-observer variability of the ABI measurement. One study evaluating inter-observer variability [49] found a standard deviation (SD) in differences in results of 0.07, suggesting that a reproducible change in ABI must be greater than 0.15 (2 SDs) to be significant. A second investigation [50] assessed 69 patients on six different days using the same technician, and found a measurement variance of 0.05. Based on these and other studies, the ABI is considered to have a reproducibility of approximately 0.10. The largest cohort to demonstrate this predominance of asymptomatic PAD was reported by Stoffers *et al.* [51] in a study performed in the Netherlands. The investigators evaluated 18 884 adults aged 45–74 years and showed a PAD prevalence of 6.9% based on an ABI < 0.95. However, only 22% of PAD patients had symptoms. The Rotterdam study [44] examined 7715 community-dwelling adults (40% men, 60% women) ≥ 55 years old. PAD diagnosis was determined using an ABI < 0.9 and claudication was diagnosed based on the WHO Rose questionnaire [52]. They found a PAD prevalence of 19.1% (16.9% in men and 20.5% in women), while claudication was present in only 1.6% (2.2% in men, 1.2% in women) of the population. Of the individuals with PAD, only 6.3% (8.7% in men, 4.9% in women) had claudication. The PAD Awareness, Risk and Treatment (PARTNERS) Study [13] focused on higher-risk individuals and evaluated 6979 primary care patients ≥ 70 years old, or 50–69 years old with a history of smoking or diabetes. As expected, the PAD prevalence was higher in this cohort (29%).

Older and frail individuals have a higher prevalence of PAD and are less likely to report symptoms due to their poor functional status. The Cardiovascular Health Study [53] found a 12% PAD prevalence among community-dwelling adults 65 years and older, and the Systolic Hypertension in the Elderly Program [42] reported a 25.5% prevalence. These two populations included healthier elderly adults. However, McDermott *et al.* [54], reporting results of an analysis among participants in the Women's Health and Aging Study (an observational study of disabled women ≥ 65 years of age living in and around Baltimore), found a PAD prevalence of 35%, of whom 63% were asymptomatic. Also, PAD prevalence reported in a study of 60 nursing home residents was 88% [55].

Other studies have used additional markers to the ABI to define the PAD population. The Edinburgh Artery Study [12] assessed PAD based on claudication among a cohort of 1592 individuals aged 55–74 years using the WHO questionnaire. They also measured ABI and added an assessment of the change in ankle systolic pressure during reactive hyperemia. The prevalence of claudication in this cohort was 4.5%, while there were 8% of the population who were asymptomatic, yet had significant impairment of blood flow to the lower extremities (ABI < 0.7 or hyperemic systolic pressure drop of > 35%; or ABI < 0.9 and hyperemic systolic pressure drop of > 20%). Criqui *et al.* [10] conducted another study to evaluate PAD prevalence among 613 adults in southern California, with an average age of 66 years. They used a series of noninvasive vascular diagnostic tests (segmental blood pressure, Doppler-derived flow velocity, post-occlusive reactive hyperemia, and pulse-reappearance half-time). They found a prevalence of PAD of 11.7%. However, the prevalence of claudication in this population was 2.2% in men and 1.7% in women.

Claudication

Many epidemiological studies have used claudication as a marker for estimating the prevalence and incidence of PAD. Many patient questionnaires have been developed to identify intermittent claudication and to distinguish it from other types of leg pain. The first to be developed for use in epidemiologic studies in 1962 was the Rose questionnaire [44], which was eventually adopted by the WHO in 1968. The initial study evaluating the reliability of this questionnaire among 37 patients with classic claudication (angiographically confirmed PAD) and 18 patients with atypical leg pain (sciatica, osteoarthritis, and calf cramps), had a 91.9% sensitivity and 100% specificity. Not surprisingly (considering prior information in this chapter), larger studies performed more recently that used ABI as a comparison found a sensitivity of 8.6% [56] and sensitivity of 91% for diagnosis of PAD. Another leg symptom detection questionnaire, the Edinburgh claudication questionnaire (ECQ) [36], was developed in 1992. Further, the San Diego claudication questionnaire (SDCQ) [57] was developed

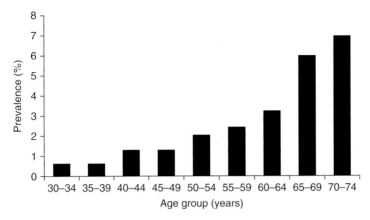

Figure 1.4 Mean prevalence of claudication in large population studies. *Source*: adapted with permission from Norgren *et al.* [19].

in 1996. The SDCQ was a revised and expanded version of the WHO/Rose questionnaire and incorporated laterality.

Overall, the estimated prevalence of claudication assessed by an intermittent claudication questionnaire ranges from 0.4% in the 30- to 34-year-olds to at least 8% in the 70- to 74-year-olds [19] (Figure 1.4). Finnish investigators in the 1960s [58] interviewed 5738 men and 5224 women aged 30–59 years and found a prevalence of claudication of 2.1% in males and 1.8% in females. Scottish investigators [59] also found similar prevalence of claudication (1.8%), while Diehm *et al.* [60] in Germany documented claudication in 2.8% of adults aged 65 and older. Ness *et al.* [61] examined and interviewed 467 and 1444 elderly men and women (mean age 80 years) in an academic outpatient geriatrics practice. They found a 20% prevalence of claudication in the men and 13% in the women. Again, it should be noted that only a minority of patients with PAD would have classic claudication. To further illustrate this, we present the prevalence of claudication against the actual prevalence of PAD in various studies (Table 1.2).

Kannel and McGee [35] examined 26-year follow-up data of the Framingham Study Cohort of 5209 subjects. They reported that 176 men and 119 women developed occlusive peripheral arterial disease manifested as claudication. They also demonstrated that the incidence of claudication increased sharply with age until 75 years of age, with about a twofold male predominance at all ages. Their findings supported the evidence that elderly people (>60 years) suffer the most from claudication. Notably, at around 50 years of age, the prevalence of claudication is thought to be about 1–2%. At > 50 years, the estimated biannual incidence of claudication is 0.7% in males and 0.4% in females.

Atypical Leg Pain

Most individuals with lower extremity PAD do not have classic (typical) claudication but may have more subtle impairments of lower extremity function. Historically the WHO Rose questionnaire and other surveys of claudication have categorized PAD patients as symptomatic (claudication) or asymptomatic. However, many individuals with PAD have leg symptoms that are not claudication but cannot be completely attributed to other etiologies. For example, leg pain may persist or be present at rest in a patient without CLI, or the patient may have difficulty distinguishing pain syndromes from other etiologies, such as lumbar disc disease, from PAD. The San Diego claudication questionnaire allowed for lateralization of leg symptoms and added an atypical category to the original leg symptom characterization by the Rose questionnaire. Hirsch *et al.* [13], employed the questionnaire among 6979 high risk patients (≥70 years or 50–69 years with history of smoking or diabetes). Among people with a new diagnosis of PAD, only 6% had claudication, 48% were asymptomatic, 46% had atypical leg pain, and only 6% had typical claudication. Among those with prior diagnosis of PAD, only 13% had claudication; 26% were asymptomatic, and 62% had atypical leg pain. One report [54] evaluated upper and lower extremity functioning in 933 women enrolled in the Women's Health and Aging Study. Among women with PAD (ABI < 0.9) in this cohort, 63% had no exertional pain. However, even these asymptomatic individuals had evidence of worse lower extremity physical function, defined by a slower walking velocity, poorer standing balance score, slower time to rise from a seated position, and fewer blocks walked per week. These findings go on to buttress the fact that individuals with atypical leg pain are at least as impaired as those with typical claudication. In our experience in clinic, we note that atypical leg pain is much more common than expected, with up to 70% of referred PAD patients having atypical symptoms or a mixture of typical and atypical features.

Critical Limb Ischemia

A chronic and severe decrease in leg perfusion may lead to CLI, defined by ischemic rest pain, non-healing wounds and gangrene. The term "CLI" has traditionally implied a high risk of amputation if leg perfusion is not improved. Yet, the true natural history of CLI is not well studied and has been indirectly (and probably inaccurately) estimated from rates of limb revascularization and ischemic amputation. In individuals over 50 years who have higher prevalence of claudication, CLI is thought to have a 1% prevalence. Among high-risk individuals the prevalence could be as high as 12%. In the highest risk group – those 70 years and older, or in those aged 50–69 years who smoke or have diabetes – the prevalence is estimated to approach 29% [13].

More objectively, in 2006, Jensen *et al.* [62] estimated CLI prevalence in Norway using a questionnaire among 20 291 men and women aged 40–69 years. CLI was defined as non-healing wounds or rest pain. They reported a CLI prevalence of 0.26% in men and 0.24% in women. More recently (2014), Nehler *et al.* [37] investigated a large US sample (about 12 million adults with health insurance) for PAD and CLI incidence and prevalence based on insurance claims between 2003 and 2008 and reported an annual CLI incidence of 0.35% and overall prevalence of 1.33%.

Acute Limb Ischemia

Acute limb ischemia is limb ischemia resulting from thrombotic, embolic, or traumatic arterial occlusion, with symptoms and signs developing over a period of two weeks or less [63]. Data for incidence of ALI are sparse. Using a survey of vascular surgeons in Great Britain and Ireland, Campbell *et al.* [64] reported 539 episodes of acute lower limb ischemia in a 3-month period. This translates to an estimated incidence of 3.7/100 000 people per year in the general UK population. Note that these data are for the lower extremity alone. The US estimate of ALI (both lower and upper extremity) was reported by Dormandy *et al.* in 1999 [65] as 14/100 000 people per year. It is important to note that ALI is a surgical emergency and that delayed treatment beyond 6 hours can lead to permanent disability. Amputation and mortality rates for ALI are 13% and 10%, respectively, and increase with delayed diagnosis and treatment [66, 67].

Risk Factors for Development of PAD

Systemic atherosclerosis is the main cause of PAD. Although it is difficult to determine the exact time of PAD incidence in a particular individual, given that it is often asymptomatic (unlike stroke, for example), the same risk factors have demonstrated an association with incident PAD in multiple studies. Further, it is also biologically plausible to assert that the same risk factors that contribute to the development and propagation of atherosclerosis in other vascular beds also lead to the initiation and worsening of PAD, although some (especially tobacco use and diabetes) are known to be most strongly associated with PAD incidence. Major PAD risk factors include age (which has been extensively covered), cigarette smoking, diabetes, hypertension, and hyperlipidemia. Others include elevated C-reactive protein (CRP) levels and hyperhomocysteinemia. Figure 1.5 [68] displays the ORs of major PAD risk factors in HICs and LMICs that were defined in a recent global report which performed a meta-analysis of the effect size of 14 risk factors that were investigated in at least three retained studies using multivariate design. We will now focus on each of the major risk factors of PAD.

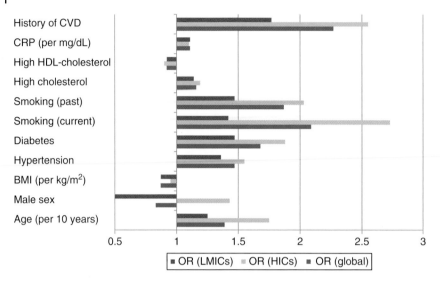

Figure 1.5 Odds ratios (ORs) of major peripheral artery disease risk factors in high-income countries (HICs) and low- to middle-income countries (LMICs). CVD, cerebrovascular disease; CRP, C-reactive protein; HDL, high-density lipoprotein; BMI, body mass index. *Source:* adapted with permission from Criqui and Aboyans [68] and Fowkes *et al.* [23].

Tobacco Use

As early as the 1970s, smoking has been recognized as an incredibly powerful risk factor for PAD [69]. Cigarette smoke causes endothelial dysfunction by reducing nitric oxide-dependent vasodilation, leading to increased atherosclerosis [70]. Analysis of the Edinburgh Artery Study [71, 72] showed that smokers are up to three times more likely to have PAD than coronary artery disease. The odds ratio for smoking in PAD ranged from 1.8 to 5.6, while that for smoking and heart disease ranged from 1.1 to 1.6. In the Framingham study [73], about 80% of individuals with claudication smoked. Smoking increases the risk of PAD by up to sevenfold [25, 51] and there also appears to be a dose–response relationship between smoking (including number of cigarettes smoked per day and number of years smoked) and PAD [72]. Secondhand smoke exposure has also been shown to lead to a 1.67-fold increased risk of developing PAD [74].

In the recent global report by Fowkes *et al.* [23], smokers had a 2.72-fold higher odds for developing PAD than non-smokers in HICs and 1.42-fold in LMICs. Ingolfsson *et al.* [33], using Poisson regression, showed in Iceland that rates of claudication dropped from 1.7/1000 per year in 1970 to 0.6/1000 per year in 1984 in younger men and from 6.0 to 2.0 in those aged 70 years and older. This drop was attributed to decreased smoking and cholesterol levels. Other studies have shown that smoking cessation leads to a reduction in claudication symptoms and mortality [75, 76]. Smoking also reduces the chances of success of surgical revascularization procedures in PAD patients and increases risk of amputation [33].

Diabetes Mellitus

The risk of claudication in diabetics has been found to be at least double that in nondiabetics [77]. Further, CLI and amputation occur up to 10 times more frequently among diabetic PAD patients than among their counterparts without diabetes [78]. In individuals without diabetes who have insulin resistance, the risk of PAD is higher than in those who do not have insulin resistance [79]. Risk is also higher among non-diabetics with hyperinsulinemia [80].

Diabetes has been shown by multiple studies to be associated with a two- to fourfold increased risk of PAD [24, 51, 53]. Hiatt *et al.* [21] showed that up to 20% of PAD patients are also diabetic; furthermore, the attributable fraction of diabetes for incident PAD was about 14% [81]. In the Framingham Heart Study [35], diabetes had an OR of 3.5 in men and 8.6 in women for risk of PAD. The longer a person has diabetes, the more likely it is that he or she will develop PAD. In one study [82], newly diagnosed diabetes had only borderline association with incident PAD. Globally, the OR of PAD in diabetics is 1.88 in HICs and 1.47 in LMICs compared with non-diabetics. Diabetics with PAD have worse outcomes and increased progression to CLI than do non-diabetics with PAD. Diabetics are up to 15 times more likely to develop CLI and undergo an amputation [83] and have a threefold higher mortality than non-diabetics with PAD [84].

Dyslipidemia

Historically, there have been conflicting reports concerning the effect of dyslipidemia on PAD risk. The Edinburgh Artery Study found an increased risk of PAD with elevated total cholesterol and a reduced risk with elevated high-density lipids (HDLs) [72]. Meijer *et al.* [44] and Newman *et al.* [53] also found a positive association between total cholesterol and PAD. In the analysis of the Framingham study by Kannel *et al.* [30] PAD risk was two times higher with cholesterol levels > 270 mg/100 mL. However, when Murabito *et al.* [25] analyzed the Framingham data using a total cholesterol threshold of 240 mg/100 mL, this relationship was attenuated. In a multivariate analysis among elderly individuals, Ness *et al.* [61] did not find a significant association between total cholesterol and PAD; neither did Hughson *et al.* [69], Zimmerman *et al.* [85], or Criqui *et al.* [79]. It is not surprising that total cholesterol is a risk factor with variable results given that low-density lipoprotein is a more significant pathological component of cholesterol. Overall, there are more studies showing a link between total cholesterol and PAD than there are that do not. Hypercholesterolemia has a population attributable fraction for PAD of 17% [81]. More recently, the global estimates for PAD risk related to hypercholesterolemia were 1.19 in HICs and 1.14 in LMICs [23].

Multiple studies, including those by Ness *et al.* [61] and Curb *et al.* [86], have confirmed the protective effect of HDLs on PAD risk. Although there is also some discrepancy in reports evaluating the link between hypertriglyceridemia and PAD, the majority [24, 25, 72] show a positive association. The Edinburgh Heart Study [72] showed only a univariate association with triglycerides.

Hypertension

Hypertension is associated with an increased risk of PAD. Studies that dichotomized hypertension as yes/no demonstrated an increase in risk of PAD ranging from 1.32-fold, as observed in the Rotterdam study [51], to 2.2- (men) and 2.8-fold (women), as observed by Ness *et al.* [61]. In the Framingham cohort, Kannel *et al.* [35] found an OR of 2.5 in men and 4.0 in women for the association of hypertension and PAD. However, in Finland, Reunanen *et al.* [15] interviewed 5738 men and 5224 women aged 30–59 years and did not find a significant association between hypertension and claudication. The most recent global report that examined PAD risk factors [23] reported that hypertension had a 1.55 (in HICs) and 1.36 (in LMICs) increased risk of PAD.

Some reports have examined systolic and diastolic blood pressure. In the report by Fowkes *et al.* [72], for each 10 mmHg rise in systolic blood pressure, there were ORs of 1.2 (univariate model) and 1.1 (multivariate model) (both significant) for claudication. There was no association between diastolic blood pressure and PAD. Other studies have corroborated the link between systolic blood pressure and PAD, and diastolic pressure does not have a significant association [51, 53]. Due to the high prevalence of hypertension, the population risk of PAD attributable to hypertension is reported as 41% [81].

Homocysteinemia

Since the 1980s [87, 88], homocysteinemia has been shown to be associated with an increased risk of PAD. In 1998, Aronow *et al.* [89] examined 147 men and women with PAD and 373 men and women without PAD with a mean age of 81 years. They found that plasma homocysteine was a significant independent risk factor for PAD with an OR of 1.13 for each 1 μmol/L increase. One meta-analysis in 1995 showed an OR of 6.8 (95% CI: 2.9–15.8) for a 5 μmol/L difference in fasting total homocysteine [90]. The OR found in this study for CAD was 1.6 for men and 1.8 for women. Another meta-analysis of 14 studies in 2009 [91] showed that homocysteine was significantly elevated, with a pooled mean difference of +4.31 μmol/L in PAD patients compared with controls. Robinson *et al.* [92] reported that homocysteine concentrations > 12.1 μmol/L are associated with a twofold increased risk of atherosclerotic vascular disease (PAD, CAD and stroke). It has been reported that up to 40% of PAD patients have elevated homocysteine levels and that the levels are even higher in those with claudication [93, 94]. Increased homocysteine levels also increase the risk of PAD progression [93]. Recently, Khandanpour *et al.* [91] evaluated the effect of folate supplementation on PAD among eight clinical trials, but there was inconsistency in the reported outcomes. However, there are no randomized studies indicating that treating homocysteine reduces progression of disease.

C-Reactive Protein and Fibrinogen

Serologic markers of inflammation associated with systemic atherosclerosis are also associated with PAD. Among healthy volunteers enrolled in the Physicians' Health Study [95], both CRP and fibrinogen were found to be significantly associated with PAD. Multivariate analyses showed ORs of 2.8 for CRP and 2.2 for fibrinogen in the upper quartile compared with the lowest quartile. In this study, CRP was highest in those who ultimately required vascular surgery. In a case–control study with 212 cases and 475 controls, all female aged ~ 50 years, Bloemenkamp *et al.* [96] found that elevated CRP levels were associated with PAD (OR = 3.1 for women in the fourth quartile compared with women in the first quartile). Among elderly individuals in the Honolulu Heart Program [86], fibrinogen had an OR of 1.28 for PAD risk.

In multivariable models adjusting for traditional cerebrovascular disease (CVD) risk factors in the MESA study [97], CRP was not significantly associated with PAD. However, other markers of inflammation, including interleukin-6 (IL-6), fibrinogen, D-dimer, and homocysteine, showed significant associations with PAD, with the highest OR being 1.29 (1.08–1.53) for IL-6.

Obesity

Although obesity is associated with an increased risk of atherosclerotic diseases, including stroke and CAD [98], it does not appear to be positively associated with PAD. In fact, most studies have shown a negative association with higher BMI related to lower PAD risk. In a cross-sectional analysis of the MESA study [97], a 1 kg/m^2 increase in body mass index (BMI) was associated with a slightly lower prevalence of PAD (OR = 0.97, 95% CI: 0.94–0.99). This was similar to findings by Newman *et al.* [53] in CHS that BMI reduced risk of PAD (OR = 0.94, 95% CI: 0.91–0.97). In the cross-sectional analysis of the Honolulu heart study [86], a 1 kg/m^2 increase in BMI also showed 36% reduced odds of PAD. However, BMI was not significantly associated with PAD in the longitudinal analysis of the same study (OR = 0.92, 95% CI: 0.76–1.11). More recently, in Fowkes *et al.*'s global meta-analysis [23], BMI used as a continuous variable (per 1 kg/m^2 increase) did not show any association with PAD. However, BMI when dichotomized (> or ≤ 25 kg/m^2) showed a reduced risk of PAD in LMICs (OR = 0·72, 95% CI: 0·63–0·81) but there was no association with PAD in HICs (OR = 0·96, 95% CI: 0·84–1·10). The overall global association was however significant (OR = 0·83, 95% CI: 0·75–0·91). In the Framingham Study [35], claudication was significantly inversely related to relative weight in men in multivariable analysis and seemed to have a U-shaped non-linear relationship with relative weight in women. One study that showed increased risk of PAD with higher BMI was conducted among over 10 000 middle-aged men in Israel [34], and reported an OR of 1.24 for incident claudication for each 5.0 kg/m^2 increase in BMI.

One possible explanation for these findings is that BMI may not be the best indicator for obesity in individuals aged 60 years and above [99]. Douketis and Sharma [100] suggested that in older people, because of loss of lean body mass, BMI can remain unchanged or even decrease although adiposity increases. One study that lends more credence to this is that conducted by Ix *et al.* [101]. In that study, the authors hypothesized that the previous findings in the BMI/PAD association may be due to lower weight among smokers and those with poor health status. In the general population of 5419 adults ≥ 65 years old, each 5-unit increase in BMI was inversely associated with PAD (prevalence ratio [PR] = 0.92, 95% CI: 0.85–1.0). However, among persons in good health who had never smoked, the direction of the association was opposite but not statistically significant (PR = 1.2, 95% CI: 0.94–1.52). When results were calculated among never smokers in good health, using BMI at 50 years old and prevalent PAD, or at baseline and incident PAD, a positive association was found – PR = 1.30, 95% CI: 1.11–1.51, and hazard ratio = 1.32, 95% CI: 1.0–1.76, respectively.

Some studies have shown that higher waist:hip ratio rather than BMI or body fat percentage is associated with higher risk of PAD [102–104], suggesting that central adiposity may be more closely related to an increased risk of PAD. More research is needed to define the true relation between obesity and PAD, but it would appear that the relationship is more likely to be U-shaped.

Other Risk Factors

Multiple non-traditional risk factors for PAD have been studied. Hypothyroidism has been shown to be associated with increased PAD risk, especially in older individuals. One study [105] in 249 men and women with a mean age of 79 years showed a significantly higher prevalence of PAD in individuals with subclinical hypothyroidism (78%) than in those who were euthyroid (17%).

Few PAD studies, including the MESA and ARIC studies, are multi-racial. These permit comparisons of the effect of race on PAD. Allison *et al.* [97] reported results from the MESA study showing an OR of PAD of 1.67 for blacks vs non-Hispanic whites. ARIC also showed a higher prevalence of PAD in blacks compared with whites (3.3% vs. 2.3% in males and 4.0% vs. 3.3% in females) [43]. Among Asians, the results from the Honolulu Heart Program suggests a lower PAD prevalence than comparable non-Hispanic whites [86].

The Strong Heart Study [106] showed prevalence estimates among Native Americans, similar to that reported in comparable non-Hispanic whites. Results from MESA [97] and the San Diego Population Study [107] suggest that PAD rates may be lower in Asians and Hispanics than in non-Hispanic whites. Hence PAD risk is highest in blacks, followed by Native Americans, non-Hispanic whites, Hispanics and Asians.

Various studies have shown conflicting results with alcohol intake and PAD. The Edinburgh Artery Study [108] showed a protective effect of alcohol in men but not in women. Although the association became non-significant after adjustment for socioeconomic class. In elderly Japanese American men in the Honolulu Heart study [86], alcohol intake was found to increase the risk of PAD (multivariate OR = 1.15, 95% CI: 1.02–1.31). Alcohol, however, had a protective effect among Native Americans in the Strong Heart Study [106]. Results from the Physicians Health Study [109] showed a protective effect of moderate alcohol intake in multivariate analysis. Interestingly, in that study, there was no association in the univariate analysis until after adjusting for smoking. This suggests that moderate alcohol use in otherwise healthy non-smokers may have a protective effect on PAD incidence.

Chronic kidney disease is associated with an increased risk of PAD [110, 111], as well as worse outcomes with PAD, including limb loss and mortality [112]. Regular physical activity has also been shown to have a protective effect on PAD with an OR of 0.51 [113]. Bowlin *et al.* [34] found that work problems, psychosocial coping mechanisms both at home and at work, anxiety (high vs. low; OR = 1.85, 95% CI: 1.29–2.65) and socioeconomic status were found to be associated with PAD. Of these, anxiety had the highest OR (1.85) for 5-year incident claudication. For people who already had PAD, McDermott *et al.* [114] showed that depressive symptoms led to worse outcomes. Poor oral health is also associated with PAD. When Navas-Acien *et al.* [115] examined over 2000 adults in the 1999–2000 National Health and Nutrition Examination Survey (NHANES), they found that elevated serum levels of lead and cadmium were associated with an increased prevalence of PAD. Hung *et al.* [116] showed that incident tooth loss was significantly associated with elevated risk of subsequent occurrence of PAD. In this study, among men with a history of periodontal diseases, tooth loss had a relative risk of 1.88 for PAD. There are also data suggesting that the presence of antiphospholipid antibodies in patients undergoing lower extremity bypass operations was a significant independent risk factor for progression of PAD [117]. Eraso *et al.* [118] found that lower circulating fetuin-A was associated with PAD in type 2 diabetes beyond traditional and novel cardiovascular risk factors. In a multivariable analysis, a 1 SD decrease in fetuin-A increased the odds of PAD (OR = 1.6, P = 0.02). Although there is evidence [119] that some of the variability in ABI could be explained by additive genetic effects, data for the genetic association of PAD have been inconsistent. However, a family history of PAD has been shown to be associated with incident PAD in multivariate analyses both in the Framingham and San Diego Population Study cohorts [120, 121].

Recently, Duval *et al.* [122] derived a risk score to detect prevalent PAD in any given population. They used data from the REACH registry and externally validated it using the Framingham Offspring Study. PAD presence was determined by a history of previous or current claudication, lower extremity arterial intervention, or ABI < 0.9. Multivariable stepwise logistic regression was used to identify cross-sectional correlates of PAD from demographic, clinical, and laboratory variables. Age, sex, smoking, diabetes, BMI, hypertension, history of heart failure, CAD, and CVD were predictive of PAD prevalence. The model-estimated PAD prevalence corresponded closely with actual PAD prevalence in each population. The C-statistic was 0.61 for derivation, 0.60 for internal validation and 0.63 for external validation when ABI < 0.9 was used, and 0.64 when clinical PAD was used. This score can be used as a tool to validate a given estimate of PAD in a population.

Awareness of PAD in the Community

Despite the high prevalence and poor cardiovascular outcomes of PAD, the general public awareness of PAD risk remains low. The National Heart, Lung, and Blood Institute partnered with the national Peripheral Artery Disease Coalition and initiated a national PAD awareness campaign – Stay in Circulation: Take Steps to Learn About PAD – in 2003. The national Peripheral Arterial Disease Coalition, coordinated by the Vascular Disease Foundation, is an alliance of > 50 cardiovascular and vascular health professional societies, health advocacy groups, and government agencies united to provide accurate health information to those with or at risk for PAD. As part of this initiative, a survey of US adults was conducted in 2006 to determine the general public awareness of PAD [123]. The survey found that 74.2% of US adults were not aware of the meaning and risk factors of PAD. What is particularly striking is that the awareness of other diseases which are much less common than PAD exceeds that of PAD. Even among those who are aware of PAD, the awareness of the consequences remains low (Figure 1.6).

Progression, Natural History, and Outcomes of PAD

Progression

A few studies have evaluated PAD progression in various populations [31, 124–129]. The lowest estimate of progression in these studies is 2.5%/year developing rest pain or gangrene [125]. In this study, PAD progressed at a rate

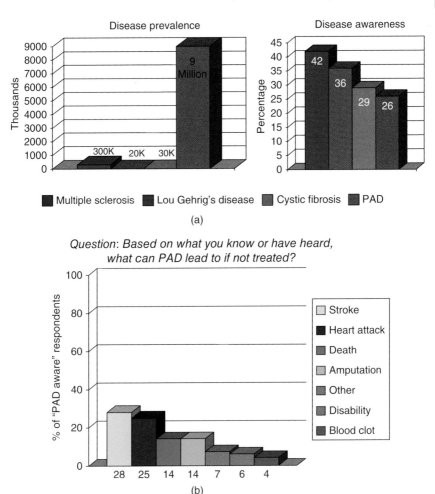

Figure 1.6 (a) Comparison of disease prevalence and the relative awareness of the general US population. (b) Perceived consequences of peripheral artery disease (PAD) among "PAD aware" individuals. *Source*: adapted from Hirsch *et al.* [123].

of around three times greater in the first year after diagnosis than in subsequent years. Using ABI and posterior tibial peak forward flow velocity, Bird *et al.* [129] found a categorical progression of 3.7%/year (16.9% over 4.6 years of follow-up). The highest reported estimate of progression is 9.1%/year [127], and this was determined based on angiographic evidence of disease progression. Given that angiography will be most accurate, we propose that one would expect a 9–10% annual progression of PAD. Two of these studies estimated the average annual change in ABI. Fowkes *et al.* [128] calculated a change of

0.01/year, while the estimate from Bird *et al.* [129] was −0.02 over a 4.6-year follow-up.

Factors that increase risk of PAD also lead to progression of already established disease. In various studies, age [31, 129], smoking and diabetes [31, 129, 130], dyslipidemia [31, 129, 130], typical claudication, PAD in the contralateral leg and previous intervention [31], lipoprotein(a) and high-sensitivity CRP [130] have been shown to be independently associated with PAD progression in various patient groups. Diabetes seems to be a stronger factor in progression of PAD in smaller lower extremity arteries [130], while hypertriglyceridemia has been shown to be particularly important in predicting progression and onset of CLI among smokers [131]. Patients who develop PAD prior to the age of 45 (premature PAD) are more likely to have faster disease progression and worse outcomes, including limb loss and mortality [132, 133]. PAD may progress, especially in the infrapopliteal arteries, without significant change in the ABI [134].

Natural History and Outcomes

The systemic nature of the atherosclerotic process also contributes to development of concomitant disease of the arteries to the heart and brain. Consequently, patients with PAD have an associated increased risk of cardiovascular ischemic events, such as MI, ischemic stroke, and death [135]. The co-prevalence of PAD with other atherosclerotic diseases has been shown in multiple studies and highlighted all through this chapter. In fact, there is an inverse correlation between ABI and odds of a major cardiovascular event. There is an abundance of evidence to show that individuals who have PAD also suffer adverse cardiovascular outcomes, including myocardial infarctions, hospitalization and stroke, at rates that are at least similar to, and often higher than, those for individuals with established coronary artery disease [136–138]. Newman *et al.* [53], in their analysis of CHS, showed that rates of MI, congestive heart failure and stroke were up to two to three times as high among individuals with PAD compared with those without. Similarly, individuals with MI, congestive heart failure and stroke had a prevalence of PAD that was 2–2.5 times the prevalence in individuals without these conditions. Figure 1.7, adapted from an analysis of the placebo arm of the Appropriate Blood Pressure Control in Diabetes study [139], depicts this. Figure 1.8 shows the co-prevalence of atherosclerotic diseases.

When compared with healthy individuals, over 15 years of follow-up, survival rates of patients with advanced PAD (CLI) are worse than those seen in patients with PAD, which in turn are worse than those for healthy individuals [19] (Figure 1.9). The frequency of systemic cardiovascular adverse events is higher than that of limb events in PAD patients [1]. This has led to PAD being recognized as a coronary heart disease risk equivalent (i.e., with PAD, there is

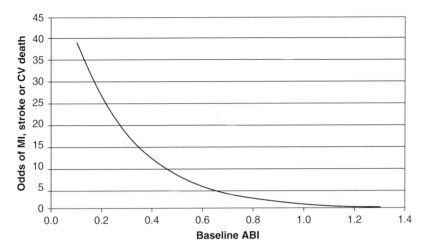

Figure 1.7 Adjusted odds of a cardiovascular event by ankle–brachial index (ABI). Data from the placebo arm of the Appropriate Blood Pressure Control in Diabetes study. CV, cardiovascular; MI, myocardial infarction. *Source*: adapted with permission from Mehler *et al.* [139].

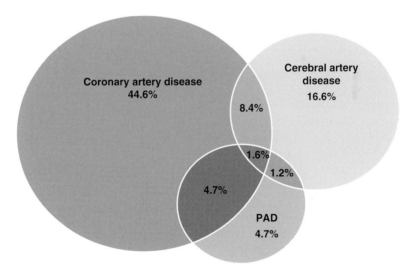

Figure 1.8 Typical overlap in vascular disease affecting different territories. Based on Reduction of Atherothrombosis for Continued Health (REACH) registry data. PAD, peripheral artery disease. *Source*: adapted with permission from Norgren *et al.* [19].

a > 20% risk of a coronary event in 10 years) in international treatment guidelines in the US and Europe [1, 140]. Figure 1.10, adapted from the ACC/AHA 2005 practice guidelines for the management of patients with peripheral

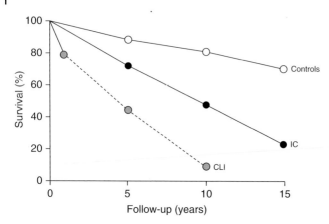

Figure 1.9 Survival of patients with peripheral arterial disease compared with healthy controls. IC, intermittent claudication; CLI, critical limb ischemia. *Source*: adapted with permission from Norgren *et al.* [19].

arterial disease (lower extremity, renal, mesenteric, and abdominal aortic) [1], summarizes the natural history of PAD.

Summary

Peripheral artery disease encompasses disorders of the structure and function of all non-coronary arteries, and specifically refers to atherosclerotic disease of lower extremity arteries. Five clinical syndromes characterize PAD. These are asymptomatic PAD, claudication, atypical leg pain, ALI and CLI.

Peripheral artery disease affects most adult populations worldwide irrespective of socioeconomic or national developmental status. The prevalence of PAD depends on what clinical syndrome defines it in a particular epidemiological study. The prevalence of claudication is lower than the prevalence of asymptomatic PAD measured by ABI. With increasing age (45–89 years), global prevalence of PAD among women ranges from 2.7% to 24.2% in HICs, and 3.96% to 18.65% in LMICs. Among men, global prevalence ranges from 2.76% to 24.77% in HICs, and 1.21% to 21.5% in LMICs.

Tobacco use, diabetes mellitus, increasing age, hypertension and hyperlipidemia are major risk factors for development and progression of PAD. Other risk factors have been described, including elevated CRP, hyperhomocysteinemia, chronic kidney disease, hypothyroidism, obesity, lower circulating fetuin-A, and periodontal disease. The systemic nature of the atherosclerotic process also contributes to development of concomitant disease of the arteries to the heart and brain. Consequently, patients with PAD have an associated increased risk of cardiovascular ischemic events (MI, stroke, and death).

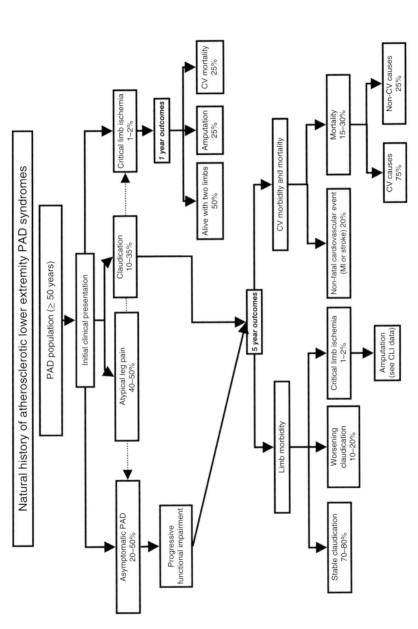

Figure 1.10 The natural history of peripheral artery disease (PAD). CV, cerebrovascular; MI, myocardial infarction; CLI, critical limb ischemia. *Source:* adapted with permission from Norgren *et al.* [19].

Despite the high prevalence and poor cardiovascular outcomes of PAD, the general public awareness of PAD risk remains low, and over 70% of US adults are not aware of the meaning and risk factors of PAD. More work needs to be done to improve awareness of PAD in the community.

References

1 Hirsch AT, Haskal ZJ, Hertzer NR, *et al.* Guidelines for the management of patients with peripheral arterial disease. J Am Coll Cardiol. 2006; 47: 1239–312.

2 Duff GL, McMillan GC. Pathology of atherosclerosis. Am J Med. 1951; 1: 92–108.

3 Li R, Duncan BB, Metcalf PA, *et al.* Atherosclerosis Risk in Communities (ARIC) Study Investigators. B-mode-detected carotid artery plaque in a general population. Stroke. 1994; 25(12): 2377–2383.

4 Kitagawa K, Hougaku H, Yamagami H, *et al.* OSACA2 Study Group. Carotid intima-media thickness and risk of cardiovascular events in high-risk patients: results of the Osaka Follow-Up Study for Carotid Atherosclerosis 2. Cerebrovasc Dis. 2007; 24(1): 35–42.

5 Cao JJ, Arnold AM, Manolio TA, *et al.* Association of carotid artery intima-media thickness, plaques, and C-reactive protein with future cardiovascular disease and all-cause mortality: the Cardiovascular Health Study. Circulation. 2007; 116(1): 32–38.

6 Hofman A, van Duijn CM, Franco OH, *et al.* The Rotterdam Study: 2012 objectives and design update. Eur J Epidemiol. 2011; 26(8): 657–686.

7 Stensland-Bugge E, Bønaa KH, Joakimsen O, Njølstad I. Sex differences in the relationship of risk factors to subclinical carotid atherosclerosis measured 15 years later: the Tromsø study. Stroke. 2000; 31(3): 574–581.

8 Joke M, Dijk, van der Graaf Y, Bots ML, *et al.* Carotid intima–media thickness and the risk of new vascular events in patients with manifest atherosclerotic disease: the SMART study. Eur Heart J. 2006; 27(16): 1971–8.

9 McGill HC Jr, Geer JC, Strong JP. Natural history of human atherosclerotic lesions. In: Sandler M, Bourne GH, eds. Atherosclerosis and Its Origin. New York: Academic Press, 1963: 39–65.

10 Criqui MH, Fronek A, Barrett-Connor E, *et al.* The prevalence of peripheral arterial disease in a defined population. Circulation. 1985; 71: 510–5.

11 McDermott MM, Fried L, Simonsick E, *et al.* Asymptomatic peripheral arterial disease is independently associated with impaired lower extremity functioning: the Women's Health and Aging Study. Circulation. 2000; 101: 1007–12.

12 Fowkes FGR, Housley E, Cawood EH, *et al.* Edinburgh Artery Study: prevalence of asymptomatic and symptomatic peripheral arterial disease in the general population. Int J Epidemiol. 1991; 20: 384–92.

13 Hirsch AT, Criqui MH, Treat-Jacobson D, *et al.* Peripheral arterial disease detection, awareness, and treatment in primary care. JAMA. 2001; 286(11): 1317–24.

14 Hiatt WR, Marshall JA, Baxter J, *et al.* Diagnostic methods for peripheral arterial disease in the San Luis Valley Diabetes Study. J Clin Epidemiol. 1990; 43: 597–606.

15 Reunanen A, Takkunen H, Aromaa A. Prevalence of intermittent claudication and its effect on mortality. Acta Med Scand. 1982; 211: 249–56.

16 McDermott MM, Mehta S, Greenland P. Exertional leg symptoms other than intermittent claudication are common in peripheral arterial disease. Arch Intern Med. 1999; 159: 387–92.

17 Criqui MH, Denenberg JO, Bird CE, *et al.* The correlation between symptoms and non-invasive test results in patients referred for peripheral arterial disease testing. Vasc Med. 1996; 1: 65–71.

18 McDermott MM, Greenland P, Liu K, *et al.* Leg symptoms in peripheral arterial disease: associated clinical characteristics and functional impairment. JAMA. 2001; 286(13): 1599–606.

19 Norgren L, Hiatt WR, Dormandy JA, *et al.* Inter-Society Consensus for the Management of Peripheral Arterial Disease (TASC II). J Vasc Surg. 2007; 45: S5–S67.

20 Creager MA, Kaufman JA, Conte MS. Clinical practice. Acute limb ischemia. N Engl J Med. 2012; 366: 2198–2206.

21 Hiatt WR, Hoag S, Hamman RF. Effect of diagnostic criteria on the prevalence of peripheral arterial disease. The San Luis Valley Diabetes Study. Circulation. 1995; 91: 1472–9.

22 Rutherford RB, Baker DJ, Ernst C, *et al.* Recommended standards for reports dealing with lower extremity ischemia: revised version. J Vasc Surg. 1997; 26: 517–38.

23 Fowkes FGR, Rudan D, Rudan I, *et al.* Comparison of global estimates of prevalence and risk factors for peripheral artery disease in 2000 and 2010: a systematic review and analysis. Lancet. 2013; 382: 1329–40.

24 Criqui MH, Denenberg JO, Langer RD, *et al.* The epidemiology of peripheral arterial disease: importance of identifying the population at risk. Vasc Med. 1997; 2: 221–6.

25 Murabito JM, D'Agostino RB, Silbershatz H, *et al.* Intermittent claudication. A risk profile from The Framingham Heart Study. Circulation. 1997; 96: 44–9.

26 Bui AL, Horwich TB, Fonarow GC. Epidemiology and risk profile of heart failure. Nat Rev Cardiol. 2011; 8(1): 30–41.

27 Chugh SS, Havmoeller R, Narayanan K, *et al.* Worldwide Epidemiology of Atrial Fibrillation: A Global Burden of Disease 2010 Study. Circulation. 2014; 129(8): 837–847.

28 Allison MA, Ho E, Denenberg JO, *et al.* Ethnic-specific prevalence of peripheral arterial disease in the United States. Am J Prev Med. 2007; 32: 328–333.

29 Eraso LH, Fukaya E, Mohler ER 3rd, *et al*. Peripheral arterial disease, prevalence and cumulative risk factor profile analysis. Eur J Prev Cardiol. 2014; 21(6): 704–11.

30 Kannel WB, Skinner JJ Jr, Schwartz MJ, *et al*. Intermittent claudication: incidence in the Framingham Study. Circulation. 1970; 41: 875–83.

31 Hooi JD, Kester ADM, Stoffers HEJH, *et al*. Incidence of and risk factors for asymptomatic peripheral arterial occlusive disease: a longitudinal study. Am J Epidemiol. 2001; 153: 666–72.

32 Kennedy M, Solomon C, Manolio TA, *et al*. Risk factors for declining ankle-brachial index in men and women 65 years or older: the Cardiovascular Health Study. Arch Intern Med. 2005; 165: 1896–902.

33 Ingolfsson IO, Sigurdsson G, Sigvaldason H, *et al*. A marked decline in the prevalence and incidence of intermittent claudication in Icelandic men 1968–1986: a strong relationship to smoking and serum cholesterol–the Reykjavik Study. J Clin Epidemiol. 1994; 47: 1237–43.

34 Bowlin SJ, Medalie JH, Flocke SA, *et al*. Epidemiology of intermittent claudication in middle-aged men. Am J Epidemiol. 1994; 140: 418–30.

35 Kannel WB, McGee DL. Update on some epidemiological features of intermittent claudication: the Framingham study. J Am Geriatr Soc. 1985; 22: 13–18.

36 Leng GC, Fowkes FG. The Edinburgh claudication questionnaire: An improved version of the WHO/Rose questionnaire for use in epidemiological surveys. J Clin Epidemiol. 1992; 45(10): 1101–9.

37 Nehler MR, Duval S, Diao L, *et al*. Epidemiology of peripheral arterial disease and critical limb ischemia in an insured national population. J Vasc Surg. 2014; 60: 686–95.

38 McDermott MM, Liu K, Criqui MH, *et al*. Ankle-brachial index and subclinical cardiac and carotid disease: the multi-ethnic study of atherosclerosis. Am J Epidemiol. 2005; 162: 33–41.

39 McDermott MM, Greenland P, Liu K, *et al*. Leg symptoms in peripheral arterial disease: associated clinical characteristics and functional impairment. JAMA. 2001; 286: 1599–1606.

40 Hirsch AT, Allison MA, Gomes AS, *et al*. American Heart Association Council on Peripheral Vascular Disease; Council on Cardiovascular Nursing; Council on Cardiovascular Radiology and Intervention; Council on Cardiovascular Surgery and Anesthesia; Council on Clinical Cardiology; Council on Epidemiology and Prevention. A call to action: women and peripheral artery disease: a scientific statement from the American Heart Association. Circulation. 2012; 125(11): 1449–72.

41 Schroll M, Munck O. Estimation of peripheral arteriosclerotic disease by ankle blood pressure measurements in a population study of 60-year-old men and women. J Chronic Dis. 1981; 34(6): 261–9.

42 Newman AB, Sutton-Tyrrell K, Vogt MT, Kuller LH. Morbidity and mortality in hypertensive adults with a low ankle/arm blood pressure index. JAMA. 1993; 270: 487–489.

43 Zheng ZJ, Sharrett AR, Chambless LE, *et al*. Associations of ankle–brachial index with clinical coronary heart disease, stroke and preclinical carotid and popliteal atherosclerosis: the Atherosclerosis Riskhin Communities (ARIC) study. Atherosclerosis. 1997; 131: 115–25.

44 Meijer WT, Hoes AW, Rutgers D, *et al*. Peripheral arterial disease in the elderly: the Rotterdam Study. Arterioscler Thromb Vasc Biol 1998; 18: 185–92.

45 Cimminiello C. PAD: Epidemiology and pathophysiology. Thromb Res. 2002; 106(6): V295–V301.

46 Halperin JL. Evaluation of patients with peripheral vascular disease. Thromb Res. 2002; 106: V303–V311.

47 Fowkes FG. The measurement of atherosclerotic peripheral arterial disease in epidemiological surveys. Int J Epidemiol. 1988; 17: 248–54.

48 Lijmer JG, Hunink MG, van den Dungen JJ, *et al*. ROC analysis of noninvasive tests for peripheral arterial disease. Ultrasound Med Biol. 1996; 22: 391–8.

49 Baker JD, Dix DE. Variability of Doppler ankle pressures with arterial occlusive disease: an evaluation of ankle index and brachial-ankle pressure gradient. Surgery. 1981; 89: 134–7.

50 Yao ST. Haemodynamic studies in peripheral arterial disease. Br J Surg. 1970; 57: 761–6.

51 Stoffers HE, Rinkens PE, Kester AD, *et al*. The prevalence of asymptomatic and unrecognized peripheral arterial occlusive disease. Int J Epidemiol. 1996; 25: 282–90.

52 Rose GA. The diagnosis of ischaemic heart pain and intermittent claudication in field surveys. Bull World Health Organ. 1962; 27: 645–58.

53 Newman AB, Siscovick DS, Manolio TA, *et al*. Ankle-arm index as a marker of atherosclerosis in the Cardiovascular Health Study.Circulation. 1993; 88: 837–45.

54 McDermott MM, Ferrucci L, Simonsick EM, *et al*. The ankle brachial index and change in lower extremity functioning over time: the Women's Health and Aging Study. J Am Geriatr Soc. 2002; 50: 238–46.

55 Cammer-Paris BE, Libow LS, Halperin JL, Mulvihill MN. The prevalence and one-year outcome of limb arterial obstructive disease in a nursing home population. J Am Geriatr Soc. 1988; 36: 607–612.

56 Newman AB, Naydeck BL, Sutton-Tyrrell K, *et al*. The role of comorbidity in the assessment of intermittent claudication in older adults. J Clin Epidemiol. 2001; 54(3): 294–300.

57 Criqui MH, Denenberg JO, Bird CE, *et al*. The correlation between symptoms and non-invasive test results in patients referred for peripheral arterial disease testing. Vasc Med. 1996; 1: 65–71.

58 A Reunanen, H Takkunen, A Aromaa. Prevalence of intermittent claudication and its effect on mortality. Acta Med Scand. 1982: 44: 249–256.

59 Smith GD, Shipley MJ, Rose G. Intermittent claudication, heart disease risk factors, and mortality. The Whitehall Study. Circulation. 1990; 82: 1925–31.

60 Diehm C, Schuster A, Allenberg JR, *et al.* High prevalence of peripheral arterial disease and co-morbidity in 6880 primary care patients: cross-sectional study. Atherosclerosis. 2004; 172(1): 95–105.

61 Ness J, Aronow WS, Ahn C. Risk factors for peripheral arterial disease in an academic hospital-based geriatrics practice. J Am Geriatr Soc. 2000; 48: 312–14.

62 Jensen SA, Vatten LJ, Myhre HO. The prevalence of chronic critical lower limb ischaemia in a population of 20, 000 subjects 40–69 years of age. Eur J Vasc Endovasc Surg. 2006; 32(1): 60–5.

63 Creager MA, Kaufman JA, Conte MS. Acute limb ischaemia. N Engl J Med. 2012; 366: 2198–206.

64 Campbell WB, Ridler BMF, Szymanska TH. Current management of acute leg ischaemia: results of an audit by the Vascular Surgical Society of Great Britain and Ireland. Br J Surg. 1998; 85: 1498–503.

65 Dormandy J, Heeck L, Vig S. Acute limb ischemia". Semin Vasc Surg. 1999; 12(2): 148–53.

66 Henke P. Contemporary management of acute limb ischaemia: factors associated with amputation and in-hospital mortality. Semin Vasc Surg. 2009; 22: 34–40.

67 Brearly S. Acute leg ischaemia. BMJ. 2013; 346: f2681.

68 Criqui MH, Aboyans B. Circ Res. 2015; 116: 1509–26.

69 WG Hughson, JI Mann, A Garrod. Intermittent claudication: prevalence and risk factors. Br Med J. 1978; 1: 1379–81.

70 Celermajer DS, Sorensen KE, Georgakopoulos D, *et al.* Cigarette smoking and associated with dose-related and potentially reversible impairment of endothelium-dependent dilation in healthy young adults. Circulation. 1993; 88: 2149–55.

71 Price JF, Mowbray PI, Lee AJ, *et al.* Relationship between smoking and cardiovascular risk factors in the development of peripheral arterial disease and coronary artery disease: Edinburgh Artery Study. Eur Heart J. 1999; 20: 344–53.

72 Fowkes FG, Housley E, Riemersma RA, *et al.* Smoking, lipids, glucose intolerance and blood pressure as risk factor for peripheral atherosclerosis compared with ischemic heart disease in the Edinburgh Artery Study. Am J Epidemiol. 1992; 135: 331–40.

73 WB Kannel, D Shurleff. The Framingham Study. Cigarettes and the development of intermittent claudication. Geriatrics. 1973; 28: 61–8.

74 He Y, Lam TH, Jiang B, *et al.*Passive smoking and risk of peripheral arterial disease and ischemic stroke in Chinese women who never smoked. Circulation. 2008; 118: 1535–40.

75 Faulkner KW, House AK, Castleden WM. The effect of cessation of smoking on the accumulative survival rates of patients with symptomatic peripheral vascular disease. Med J Aust. 1983; 1: 217–9.

76 Jonason T, Bergström R. Cessation of smoking in patients with intermittent claudication. Effects on the risk of peripheral vascular complications, myocardial infarction and mortality. Acta Med Scand. 1987; 221: 253–60.

77 Brand FN, Abbott RD, Kannel WB. Diabetes, intermittent claudication and risk of cardiovascular events. The Framingham Study. Diabetes. 1989; 38: 504–9.

78 J Dormandy, L Heeck, S Vig. Predicting which patients will develop chronic critical leg ischemia. Semin Vasc Surg. 1999; 12: 138–41.

79 Criqui MH, Browner D, Fronek A, *et al.* Peripheral arterial disease in large vessels is epidemiologically distinct from small vessel disease: an analysis of risk factors. Am J Epidemiol. 1989; 129: 1110–19.

80 Price JF, Lee AJ, Fowkes FG. Hyperinsulinemia: a risk factor for peripheral arterial disease in a non diabetic general population. J Cardiovasc Risk. 1996; 3: 501–5.

81 Joosten MM, Pai JK, Bertoia ML, *et al.* Associations between conventional cardiovascular risk factors and risk of peripheral artery disease in men. JAMA. 2012; 308: 1660–7.

82 Beks PJ, Mackaay AJ, de Neeling JN, *et al.* Peripheral arterial disease in relation to glycaemic level in an elderly Caucasian population: the Hoorn study. Diabetologia. 1995; 38: 86–96.

83 Most RS, Sinnock P. The epidemiology of lower extremity amputations in diabetic individuals. Diabetes Care. 1983; 6: 87–91.

84 Jude EB, Oyibo SO, Chalmers N, Boulton AJ. Peripheral arterial disease in diabetic and nondiabetic patients: a comparison of severity and outcome. Diabetes Care. 2001; 24: 1433–7.

85 Zimmerman BR, Palumbo PJ, Fallon WM, *et al.* A prospective study of peripheral occlusive arterial disease in diabetes: III. Initial lipid and lipoprotein findings. Mayo Clinic Proc. 1981; 56: 233–42.

86 Curb JD, Masaki K, Rodriguez BL, *et al.* Peripheral artery disease and cardiovascular risk factors in the elderly. The Honolulu Heart Program. Arterioscler Thromb Vasc Biol. 1996; 16: 1495–1500.

87 Boers GHJ, Smals AGH, Trijbels FJM, *et al.* Heterozygosity for homocystinuria in premature peripheral and cerebral occlusive arterial disease. N Engl J Med. 1985; 313: 709–15.

88 Malinow MR, Kang SS, Taylor IM, *et al.* Prevalence of hyperhomocyst(e) inemia in patients with peripheral arterial occlusive disease. Circulation. 1989; 79: 1180–8.

89 Aronow WS, Ahn C. Association between plasma homocysteine and peripheral arterial disease in older persons. Coronary Artery Dis. 1998; 9: 49–50.

90 Boushey CJ, Beresford SA, Omenn GS, Motulsky AG. A quantitative assessment of plasma homocysteine as a risk factor for vascular disease. Probable benefits of increasing folic acid intakes. JAMA. 1995; 274: 1049–57.

91 Khandanpour N, Loke YK, Meyer FJ, *et al*. Homocysteine and peripheral arterial disease: systematic review and meta-analysis. Eur J Vasc Endovasc Surg. 2009; 38: 316–22.

92 Robinson K, Arheart K, Refsum H, *et al*. Low circulating folate and vitamin B6 concentrations: risk factors for stroke, peripheral vascular disease, and coronary artery disease. European COMAC Group. Circulation. 1998; 97: 437–43. (Erratum in: Circulation 1999; 99: 983.)

93 Taylor LM Jr, DeFrang RD, Harris EJ Jr, *et al*. The association of elevated plasma homocyst(e)ine with progression of symptomatic peripheral arterial disease. J Vasc Surg. 1991; 13: 128–36.

94 Molgaard J, Malinow MR, Lassvik C, *et al*. Hyperhomocyst(e)inaemia: an independent risk factor for intermittent claudication. J Intern Med. 1992; 231: 273–9.

95 Ridker PM, Stampfer MJ, Rifai N. Novel risk factors for systemic atherosclerosis: a comparison of C-reactive protein, fibrinogen, homocysteine, lipoprotein(a), and standard cholesterol screening as predictors of peripheral arterial disease. JAMA. 2001; 285: 2481–5.

96 Bloemenkamp DG, van den Bosch MA, Mali WP, *et al*. Novel risk factors for peripheral arterial disease in young women. Am J Med. 2002; 113: 462–467.

97 Allison MA, Criqui MH, McClelland RL, *et al*. The effect of novel cardiovascular risk factors on the ethnic-specific odds for peripheral arterial disease in the Multi-Ethnic Study of Atherosclerosis (MESA). J Am Coll Cardiol. 2006; 48: 1190–7.

98 Poirier P, Giles TD, Bray GA, *et al*. Obesity and cardiovascular disease: pathophysiology, evaluation, and effect of weight loss: an update of the 1997 American Heart Association Scientific Statement on Obesity and Heart Disease from the Obesity Committee of the Council on Nutrition, Physical Activity, and Metabolism. Circulation. 2006; 113: 898–918.

99 Kyle UG, Genton L, Hans D, *et al*. Total body mass, fat mass, fat-free mass, and skeletal muscle in older people: cross-sectional differences in 60-year-old persons. J Am Geriatr Soc. 2001; 49: 1633–1640.

100 Douketis JD, Sharma AM. Obesity and cardiovascular disease: pathogenic mechanisms and potential benefits of weight reduction. Semin Vasc Med. 2005; 5: 25–33.

101 Ix JH, Biggs ML, Kizer JR, Mukamal KJ, Djousse L, *et al*. Association of body mass index with peripheral arterial disease in older adults: the Cardiovascular Health Study. Am J Epidemiol. 2011; 174: 1036–43.

102 Lu B, Zhou J, Waring ME, Parker DR, Eaton CB. Abdominal obesity and peripheral vascular disease in men and women: a comparison of

waist-to-thigh ratio and waist circumference as measures of abdominal obesity. Atherosclerosis. 2010; 208: 253–7.

103 Vogt MT, Cauley JA, Kuller LH, Hulley SB. Prevalence and correlates of lower extremity arterial disease in elderly women. Am J Epidemiol. 1993; 137: 559–68.

104 Katsilambros NL, Tsapogas PC, Arvanitis MP, *et al.* Risk factors for lower extremity arterial disease in non-insulin-dependent diabetic persons. Diabet Med. 1996; 13: 243–2.

105 Mya MM, Aronow WS. Increased prevalence of peripheral arterial disease in older men and women with subclinical hypothyroidism. J Gerontol A Biol Sci Med Sci. 2003; 58A: M68–9.

106 Fabsitz RR, Sidawy AN, Go O, *et al.* Prevalence of peripheral arterial disease and associated risk factors in American Indians: the Strong Heart Study. Am J Epidemiol. 1999; 149: 330–8.

107 Criqui MH, Vargas V, Denenberg JO, *et al.* Ethnicity and peripheral arterial disease: the San Diego Population Study. Circulation. 2005; 112: 2703–7.

108 Jepson RG, Fowkes FG, Donnan PT, Housley E. Alcohol intake as a risk factor for peripheral arterial disease in the general population in the Edinburgh Artery Study. Eur J Epidemiol. 1995; 11: 9–14.

109 Camargo CA Jr, Stampfer MJ, Glynn RJ, *et al.* Prospective study of moderate alcohol consumption and risk of peripheral arterial disease in US male physicians. Circulation. 1997; 95: 577–80.

110 Rajagopalan S, Dellegrottaglie S, Furniss AL, *et al.* Peripheral arterial disease in patients with end-stage renal disease: observations from the Dialysis Outcomes and Practice Patterns Study (DOPPS). Circulation. 2006; 114: 1914–22.

111 O'Hare A, Johansen K. Lower-extremity peripheral arterial disease among patients with end-stage renal disease. J Am Soc Nephrol. 2001; 12: 2838–47.

112 Asqualini L, Schillaci G, Pirro M, *et al.* Renal dysfunction predicts long-term mortality in patients with lower extremity arterial disease. J Intern Med. 2007; 262: 668–77.

113 Asgeirsdóttir LP, Agnarsson U, Jónsson GS. Lower extremity blood flow in healthy men: effect of smoking, cholesterol, and physical activity – a Doppler study. Angiology. 2001; 52: 437–45.

114 McDermott MM, Greenland P, Guralnik JM, *et al.* Depressive symptoms and lower extremity functioning in men and women with peripheral arterial disease. J Gen Intern Med. 2003; 18: 461–7.

115 Navas-Acien A, Selvin E, Sharrett AR, *et al.* Lead, cadmium, smoking, and increased risk of peripheral arterial disease. Circulation. 2004; 109: 3196–201.

116 Hung HC, Willett W, Merchant A, *et al.* Oral health and peripheral arterial disease. Circulation. 2003; 107: 1152–7.

117 Lam EY, Taylor LM Jr, Landry GJ, *et al.* Relationship between antiphospholipid antibodies and progression of lower extremity arterial occlusive disease after lower extremity bypass operations. J Vasc Surg. 2001; 33: 976–82.

118 Eraso LH, Ginwala N, Qasim AN, *et al.* Association of lower plasma fetuin-a levels with peripheral arterial disease in type 2 diabetes. Diabetes Care. 2010; 33(2): 408–10.

119 Carmelli D, Fabsitz RR, Swan GE, *et al.* Contribution of genetic and environmental influences to ankle-brachial blood pressure index in the NHLBI Twin Study. National Heart, Lung, and Blood Institute. Am J Epidemiol. 2000; 151: 452–8.

120 Prushik SG, Farber A, Gona P, *et al.* Parental intermittent claudication as risk factor for claudication in adults. Am J Cardiol. 2012; 109: 736–41.

121 Wassel CL, Loomba R, Ix JH, *et al.* Family history of peripheral artery disease is associated with prevalence and severity of peripheral artery disease: the San Diego population study. J Am Coll Cardiol. 2011; 58: 1386–92.

122 Duval S, Massaro JM, Jaff MR, *et al.* REACH Registry Investigators. An evidence-based score to detect prevalent peripheral artery disease (PAD). Vasc Med. 2012; 17(5): 342–51.

123 Hirsch AT, Murphy TP, Lovell MB, *et al.* Gaps in public knowledge of peripheral arterial disease: the first national PAD public awareness survey. Circulation. 2007; 116(18): 2086–94.

124 Hess H, Mietaschk A, Deichsel G. Drug-induced inhibition of platelet function delays progression of peripheral occlusive arterial disease: a prospective double-blind arteriographically controlled trial. Lancet. 1985; i: 415–19.

125 Jelnes R, Gaardsting O, Hougaard Jensen K, *et al.* Fate in intermittent claudication: outcome and risk factors. Br Med J. 1986; 293: 1137–40.

126 Osmundson PJ, O'Fallon WM, Zimmerman BR, *et al.* Course of peripheral occlusive arterial disease in diabetes: vascular laboratory assessment. Diabetes Care. 1990; 13: 143–52.

127 Walsh DB, Gilbertson JJ, Zwolack RM, *et al.* The natural history of superficial femoral artery stenoses. J Vasc Surg. 1991; 14: 299–304.

128 Fowkes FG, Lowe GD, Housley E, *et al.* Cross-linked fibrin degradation products, progression of peripheral arterial disease, and risk of coronary heart disease. Lancet. 1993; 342: 84–6.

129 Bird CE, Criqui MH, Fronek A, *et al.* Quantitative and qualitative progression of peripheral arterial disease by non-invasive testing. Vasc Med. 1999; 4: 15–21.

130 Aboyans V, Criqui MH, Denenberg JO, *et al.* Risk factors for progression of peripheral arterial disease in large and small vessels. Circulation. 2006; 113: 2623–9.

131 Smith I, Franks PJ, Greenhalgh RM, *et al.* The influence of smoking cessation and hypertriglyceridaemia on the progression of peripheral arterial disease and the onset of critical ischaemia. Eur J Vasc Endovasc Surg. 1996; 11: 402–8.

132 Pairolero PC, Joyce JW, Skinner CR, *et al*. Lower limb ischemia in young adults: prognostic implications. J Vasc Surg. 1984; 1: 459–64.

133 Levy PJ, Hornung CA, Haynes JL, Rush DS. Lower extremity ischemia in adults younger than forty years of age: a community-wide survey of premature atherosclerotic arterial disease. J Vasc Surg. 1994; 19(5): 873–81.

134 Mohler ER 3rd, Bundens W, Denenberg J, *et al*. Progression of asymptomatic peripheral artery disease over 1 year. Vasc Med. 2012; 17(1): 10–16.

135 Criqui MH, Langer RD, Fronek A, *et al*. Mortality over a period of 10 years in patients with peripheral arterial disease. N Engl J Med. 1992; 326: 381–6.

136 Heart Protection Study Collaborative Group. MRC/BHF Heart Protection Study of cholesterol lowering with simvastatin in 20, 536 high-risk individuals: a randomised placebo controlled trial. Lancet. 2002; 360: 7–22.

137 Joint National Committee on Prevention, Detection, Evaluation, and Treatment of High Blood Pressure. The Seventh Report. NIH publication No. 04-5230. Bethesda, MD: National Institutes of Health, 2004.

138 Steg G, Bhatt DL, Wilson PWF, *et al*. for the REACH Registry Investigators. One-year cardiovascular event rates in outpatients with atherothrombosis. JAMA. 2007; 297: 1197–206.

139 Mehler PS, Coll JR, Estacio R, *et al*. Intensive blood pressure control reduces the risk of cardiovascular events in patients with peripheral arterial disease and type 2 diabetes. Circulation. 2003; 107: 753–6.

140 National Cholesterol Education Program (NCEP) Expert Panel on Detection, Evaluation, and Treatment of High Blood Cholesterol in Adults: Third Report of the National Cholesterol Education Program (NCEP) Expert Panel on Detection, Evaluation, and Treatment of High Blood Cholesterol in Adults (Adult Treatment Panel III): Final Report. NIH publication No. 02-5215. Bethesda, MD: National Institutes of Health; 2002.

2

Office Evaluation of Peripheral Artery Disease – History and Physical Examination Strategies

Maen Nusair[1] and Robert S. Dieter[2]

[1] *PeaceHealth Southwest Heart and Vascular Center, Vancouver, WA, USA*
[2] *Loyola University Medical Center, Maywood, IL, USA*

Introduction

The prevalence of peripheral artery disease (PAD) is estimated to be 3–13% worldwide and is a major cause of morbidity and mortality in affected individuals [1]. It is also a marker of systemic atherosclerosis. Careful history and physical examination allow for early diagnosis and implementation of interventions to modify the risk of morbidity and mortality.

The effective medical interview allows for the exchange of pertinent information in addition to building a therapeutic alliance with the patient. The diagnosis of PAD can be identified on the basis of a good medical history. If leg discomfort is not clearly vascular in origin, a differential diagnosis can be formulated and then further narrowed down by thoughtful physical examination.

Identifying At-Risk Individuals

Multiple risk factors for PAD have been identified. It is important to identify the presence of these risk factors in each patient not only for risk assessment for PAD but also for risk modification.

The National Health and Nutrition Examination Survey (NHANES) in the United States found that an ankle–brachial index (ABI) ≤ 0.90 was more common in non-Hispanic blacks (7.8%) than in whites (4.4%) [2]. This difference was independent of traditional risk factors [3]. The prevalence of PAD increases with age in both men and women progressively after the age of 40 years. The prevalence of PAD, according to NHANES, is about 0.9% in individuals between the ages 40–49 years. The prevalence increases to 23.3% in individuals over 80 years of age [4].

According to the NHANES data, current smoking is associated with an increased risk of PAD (odds ratio = 3.39) [5]. Furthermore, a diagnosis of PAD is made approximately a decade earlier in smokers than in non-smokers. The severity of PAD tends to increase with the number of cigarettes smoked [2]. The Edinburgh Artery Study found a decreased risk of claudication for patients who stopped smoking compared with those who continued to smoke [6].

Diabetics are at an increased risk for PAD. It is estimated that for every 1% increase in hemoglobin A1c, there is a corresponding 26% increased risk of PAD [7]. In the Framingham study, a fasting total cholesterol level 270 mg/dL was associated with a doubling of the incidence of intermittent claudication, and for each 40 mg/dL increase in total serum cholesterol, the odds of developing symptomatic PAD increased by 1.2 [8]. Statin therapy was shown to decrease vascular mortality by 17% [9].

Regional Symptom Analysis

Neurologic Symptoms

Cerebrovascular accidents in the form of transient ischemic attack (TIA) or stroke are frequently a manifestation of vascular disease. TIA is defined as a transient episode of neurologic dysfunction caused by focal brain, spinal cord, or retinal ischemia, without acute infarction. Ischemic stroke is, on the other hand, defined as infarction of central nervous system tissue. This definition, which is endorsed by the 2009 guidelines of the American Heart Association and American Stroke Association (AHA/ASA), is a departure from the classic definition of TIA focal neurologic symptom and/or sign lasting less than 24 hours. This tissue-centric definition emphasizes that there is a risk of permanent tissue injury (i.e., infarction) even when the focal neurologic symptoms are transient [10]. The specific neurologic deficits can typically be categorized as anterior circulation or posterior circulation events (Figure 2.1) [11].

Amaurosis fugax, or transient monocular blindness, occurs when a plaque travels from the proximal aorta or internal carotid artery to the ipsilateral ophthalmic artery. Patients will frequently report monocular vision loss that begins as haziness in the upper fields and progresses downward, like "a veil" or "a shade being drawn." The vision loss usually only lasts for a few seconds or minutes [12]. When amaurosis fugax is secondary to carotid artery disease, the annual risk of stroke is estimated to be 2–3% [13].

The vertebral arteries normally originate from the proximal subclavian arteries, as such disease of the subclavian or innominate arteries proximal to the

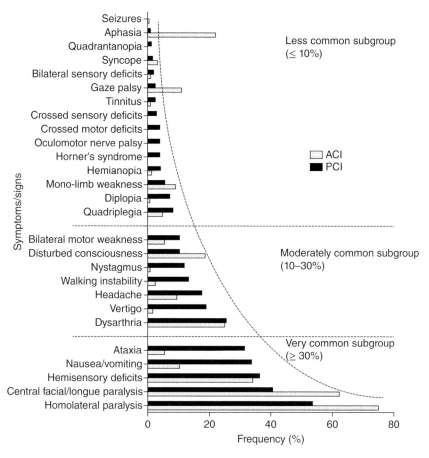

Figure 2.1 Posterior versus anterior stroke symptom. ACI, anterior circulation infarction; PCI, posterior circulation infarction. *Source*: Tao *et al.* [11].

vertebral artery origin can cause reduction of vertebral artery flow. Subclavian steal refers to a phenomenon of flow reversal in the vertebral artery ipsilateral to a hemodynamically significant stenosis or occlusion of the subclavian artery [14]. One-third of patients with subclavian stenosis develop exercise-induced arm pain, fatigue, coolness, paresthesias, or numbness. When vertebrobasilar insufficiency develops, patients may experience vertigo, ataxia, disequilibrium, tinnitus, or hearing loss. These symptoms can be provoked by the Dieter test: by inflating a blood pressure cuff on the affected extremity and then deflating it rapidly, a hyperemic response develops in the affected upper extremity and may result in an increase in the vertebral flow reversal and bring out posterior circulation symptoms [15].

Thoracic Symptoms

When evaluating a patient with chest pain, vascular etiologies should always be considered in the differential diagnosis. A detailed history helps to differentiate this from other causes of chest pain such as cardiac causes.

Thoracic aortic aneurysms are frequently asymptomatic and diagnosed incidentally on imaging tests performed for unrelated reasons. Symptoms can arise, however, when an aneurysm expands enough to cause compression or distortion of other intrathoracic structures, erosion into adjacent bone, or symptoms related to acute complications, such as aortic dissection, or rupture. Compression of the trachea may result in wheezing, dyspnea, or cough. Dysphagia may develop secondary to esophageal compression ("dysphagia aortica"). Hemoptysis may be a sign of tracheobronchial erosion by the aneurysm. Moreover, patients with aortic root dilatation may present with symptoms of heart failure as a result of aortic valve regurgitation.

Vascular rings are congenital anomalies in the aortic arch, which result in compression of the tracheobronchial tree and/or esophagus. A complete vascular ring is said to be present when both of these structures are compressed, whereas an incomplete vascular ring is present when only one of the structures is compressed. Presenting symptoms may include stridor, wheezing and dysphagia. Dysphagia lusoria is a term used to describe dysphagia as a consequence of vascular compression of the esophagus by an anomalous right subclavian artery (arteria lusoria), causing posterior esophageal compression. Around 30–40% of patients develop dysphagia as a consequence, with the majority presenting with solid bolus dysphagia [16].

Patients with an aortic dissection typically present with severe, sharp or "tearing" chest or back pain. The pain is typically sudden and intense from onset as opposed to the crescendo pain of myocardial ischemia. The site of the pain is often indicative of the site of dissection. Anterior chest pain is typical in ascending aorta dissection; neck and jaw pain may indicate dissection involving the arch and carotid arteries. Dissection of the descending aorta causes tearing interscapular pain.

Dissection of the ascending aorta may also result in development of acute aortic regurgitation; aortic rupture into pericardial sac or pleural space may also develop, causing hypotension and shock. Extension of dissection into coronary arteries, causing myocardial ischemia and infarction, occurs in about 11% of patients with dissection of the ascending aorta, with the majority of cases involved the right coronary artery [17]. Focal neurologic symptoms, including limb paresthesia and weakness, may develop when central nervous system perfusion is affected as a result of carotid, vertebral or spinal artery involvement. Limb ischemia or mesenteric ischemia suggests compromise of their respective arterial supplies. Symptoms can also develop as a result of organ compression by an expanding hematoma. Dyspnea suggests tracheal or bronchus compression, dysphagia results from esophageal compression, and hoarseness indicates recurrent laryngeal nerve compression. A superior vena cava syndrome may be precipitated by compression of the superior vena cava.

Abdominal Pain

A complaint of abdominal pain is relatively non-specific and can be due to a variety of non-vascular causes. Clinicians should always maintain a high index of suspicion for vascular causes of abdominal pain, given the potentially devastating consequences if not diagnosed promptly and accurately.

Pain related to an abdominal aortic aneurysm (AAA) is typically located in the abdomen, with aneurysms positioned more proximally producing upper abdominal/back pain and distal aneurysms producing lower abdominal/pelvic pain or radiculopathy [18]. Pain related to an unruptured AAA is typically a vague and indolent pain, which results from compression of adjacent structures or aneurysm expansion [3].

Inflammatory AAA accounts for 5–10% of all cases of AAA and typically involves infrarenal portion of the abdominal aorta [19]. The inflammatory variant is more common in male smokers, and patients are younger and usually symptomatic, primarily from back or abdominal pain. Marked thickening of the aneurysm wall, fibrosis of the adjacent retroperitoneum, and rigid adherence of the adjacent structures to the anterior aneurysm wall characterize the inflammatory variant [19]. Immunoglobulin-4 (IgG4)-related disease has been recognized as one of the causes of inflammatory aortitis and aortic aneurysms. The exact nature and pathogenesis of this disorder remain elusive [20]. The hallmarks of IgG4-related disease are lymphoplasmacytic tissue infiltration with predominance of IgG4-positive plasma cells and T-lymphocytes, usually accompanied by fibrosis, obliterative phlebitis, and elevated serum levels of IgG4. In one study, IgG4-related AAA was present in 5% of total surgical AAA cases, and 57% of inflammatory AAA [21].

The presentation of AAA rupture is typically dramatic and is influenced by the location of the rupture, and whether the rupture is contained or free. Proximal AAA rupture near the renal arteries leads to severe back or flank pain, whereas distal AAA rupture is more likely to cause lower abdominal or pelvic pain. AAA ruptures posteriorly into the retroperitoneal cavity in approximately 80% of patients, and anteriorly into the peritoneal cavity in approximately 20% [18]. This results in development of retroperitoneal hematoma, which triggers back pain. The retroperitoneal hematoma may contain the rupture and so patients may have a subacute presentation. Anterior AAA rupture, on the other hand, results in diffuse abdominal pain and rapid hemodynamic collapse.

Mesenteric ischemia and infarction are important considerations in older adult patients presenting with abdominal pain. Mesenteric ischemia can be acute, resulting in bowel infarction, or it may present as indolent chronic abdominal pain. Chronic mesenteric ischemia may be manifested by a variety of symptoms, including abdominal pain after eating ("intestinal angina", forcing patients to avoid food), weight loss, nausea, vomiting, and diarrhea. The typical patient has a history of smoking and underlying atherosclerotic vascular disease, with approximately half of patients having known peripheral arterial disease or coronary artery disease [22]. Acute mesenteric ischemia secondary to embolism or thrombosis typically presents as rapid onset of severe periumbilical abdominal pain, which is often out of proportion to findings on physical examination. Nausea and vomiting are also common associated symptoms. Patient who develop acute mesenteric ischemia secondary to mesenteric vein thrombosis have a more insidious onset with symptoms that may have been present for days to weeks before diagnosis.

Extremity Pain

Peripheral artery disease has a wide clinical spectrum of presentation, ranging from asymptomatic disease to rest pain and ischemia-related tissue loss. The Fontaine and Rutherford classifications are used to classify PAD into different stages and categories, which aids in objectively describing the clinical disease and its course (Table 2.1). Claudication is a reproducible discomfort in a particular muscle group brought on by exercise and is relieved with rest. It is important to note that the description of discomfort is variable and may include cramping, tightness, burning, weakness, heaviness, or fatigue. Symptomatic PAD patients have variable degree of functional disability. The walking impairment questionnaire is an important semi-objective method to quantify the functional impairment. It is the most specific questionnaire for documenting the qualitative deficits of the patient with claudication while providing strong relationships with the quantitative measures of arterial disease [23] (Figure 2.2).

Table 2.1 Classification of peripheral arterial disease: Fontaine's stages and Rutherford's categories.

Fontaine		Rutherford	
Stage	Claudication	Category	Claudication
I	Asymptomatic	0	Asymptomatic
IIa	Mild	1	Mild
IIb	Moderate to severe	2	Moderate
III	Ischemic rest pain	3	Severe
IV	Ulceration or gangrene	4	Ischemic rest pain
		5	Minor tissue loss
		6	Major tissue loss

1. *Please place a ✓ in the box that best describes how much difficulty you have had walking due to pain, aches, or cramps during the last week. The response options range from "No difficulty" to "Great Difficulty."*

During the last week, *how much difficulty have you had walking due to:*	**No Difficulty**	**Slight Difficulty**	**Some Difficulty**	**Much Difficulty**	**Great Difficulty**
a. Pain, aching, or cramps in your calves?	☐ 1	☐ 2	☐ 3	☐ 4	☐ 5
b. Pain, aching, or cramps in your buttocks?	☐ 1	☐ 2	☐ 3	☐ 4	☐ 5

For the following questions, the response options range from "No Difficulty" to "Unable to Do." If you **cannot physical perform** a specified activity, for example walk 2 blocks without stopping to rest because of symptoms such as leg pain or discomfort, please place a ✓ in the box labeled "Unable to Do."

However, if you **do not perform** an activity for reasons unrelated to your circulation problems, such as climbing a flight of stairs because your home is one level or your apartment has an elevator, please place a ✓ in the box labeled "Don't Do for Other Reasons."

2. *Please place a ✓ in the box that best describes how hard it was for you to walk on level ground without stopping to rest for each of the following distances during the last week.*

During the last week, *how difficult was it for you to:*	**No Difficulty**	**Slight Difficulty**	**Some Difficulty**	**Much Difficulty**	**Unable to Do**	**Did not Do for Other Reasons**
a. Walk indoors, such as around your home?	☐ 1	☐ 2	☐ 3	☐ 4	☐ 5	☐ 6
b. Walk 50 feet?	☐ 1	☐ 2	☐ 3	☐ 4	☐ 5	☐ 6
c. Walk 150 feet? (1/2 block)?	☐ 1	☐ 2	☐ 3	☐ 4	☐ 5	☐ 6
d. Walk 300 feet? (1 block)?	☐ 1	☐ 2	☐ 3	☐ 4	☐ 5	☐ 6
e. Walk 600 feet? (2 blocks)?	☐ 1	☐ 2	☐ 3	☐ 4	☐ 5	☐ 6
f. Walk 900 feet? (3 blocks)?	☐ 1	☐ 2	☐ 3	☐ 4	☐ 5	☐ 6
g. Walk 1500 feet? (5 blocks)?	☐ 1	☐ 2	☐ 3	☐ 4	☐ 5	☐ 6

Figure 2.2 Walking distance questionnaire. *Source*: Coyne *et al.* [24].

Although PAD is progressive in the pathological sense, its clinical course as far as the leg is concerned is stable in most patients. This symptomatic stabilization may be due to the development of collaterals, metabolic adaptation of ischemic muscle, or the patient altering his or her gait to favor non-ischemic muscle groups. Around 25% of patients with claudication deteriorate in terms of clinical stage; this is most frequent during the first year after diagnosis (7%–9%) compared with 2–3% per year thereafter [2]. It is important for the clinician to specifically ask the patient about the clinical stability of the symptoms. Often this can be documented with the initial claudication distance (distance at which the patient first experiences pain with exertion) and absolute claudication distance (distance at which the patient can no longer ambulate).

End-stage PAD presents as critical limb ischemia which is said to be present when the patient develops chronic ischemic rest pain or tissue loss in the form of ulcers or gangrene. Often patients will provide a history of progressive claudication symptoms. Ischemic rest pain is classically described as stabbing, burning, or stinging, and can be associated with coldness, numbness, or parasthesias of the toes. It typically occurs at while sleeping when the limb is no longer in a dependent position. The pain is localized in the distal part of the foot or in the vicinity of an ischemic ulcer or gangrenous toe. The pain often wakes the patients at night and forces them to rub the foot, get up, or take a short walk around the room. Partial relief may be obtained by the dependent position. [2]

Unlike chronic critical limb ischemia, acute limb ischemia can develop secondary to embolus or arterial thrombosis. It is also important to recognize that acute arterial injury complicating endovascular procedures has become a more frequent cause of acute extremity ischemia. Patients classically demonstrate the six Ps: pain, pallor, pulselessness, parasthesia, poikilothermia, and paralysis. Pain associated with acute ischemia is usually located distally in the extremity, progressively increases in severity, and progresses proximally. A sudden and dramatic development of these ischemic symptoms in a previously asymptomatic patient suggests an embolic etiology, whereas rapidly worsening symptoms in a patient with chronic claudication is suggestive of arterial thrombosis.

The location of the discomfort provides the earliest clue regarding which arterial system end level is compromised. In the lower extremities, buttock and hip pain suggests aorto-iliac disease, pain in the upper two-thirds of the calf suggests superficial femoral artery, pain in the lower one-third of the calf suggests popliteal artery disease, and foot claudication should raise suspicion of tibial or peroneal artery disease.

Skin Manifestations

Skin is a highly vascular organ and thus patients with vascular disease will often have cutaneous manifestations. Patients with chronic PAD will frequently complain of cool skin, paresthesia and skin ulcers over the ischemic extremity.

Raynaud phenomenon (RP) most often affects the fingers but may also affect the toes. A typical episode is characterized by the sudden onset of cold digits in association with sharply demarcated color changes of skin pallor (white attack) or cyanotic skin (blue attack). With rewarming, the skin blushes and the erythema of reperfusion develops. The index, middle, and ring fingers are the most frequently involved digits, while the thumb is often spared entirely. Involvement of the thumb may indicate a secondary cause of RP [25]. Primary RP occurs in otherwise healthy individuals with female predominance. This phenomena can also be secondary to a variety of disorders which disrupt the normal regulation of regional blood flow to the digits and skin, such as scleroderma, systemic lupus erythematosus and other connective tissue diseases. The repetitive use of vibrating tools is also linked to secondary RP.

Hypothenar hammer syndrome classically occurs in men with a mean age of 40 years and develops in occupational settings where the worker uses the hypothenar portion of the hand as a tool to hammer, push or squeeze hard objects [26]. This syndrome develops as a result of repetitive blunt trauma. The superficial palmar branch of the ulnar artery can develop intimal damage, producing vasospasm and encouraging platelet aggregation and thrombus formation. If the damage spreads through the media into the arterial wall, aneurysm formation can occur as well. Microemboli may develop and result in digital ischemia. It is hypothesized that a thrombosed artery segment may act as a disease plexus, initiating reflexes that lead to peripheral vasospasm [26]. Neurologic symptoms such as paresthesias and pain may also result from compression of the sensory branches of the ulnar nerve which run in close proximity to the ulnar artery [26].

Acrocyanosis is a disorder, which typically causes symmetrical painless blue discoloration of the hands or feet. It is aggravated by cold exposure and is often associated with hyperhidrosis of hands and feet. Patient with acrocyanosis do not experience the sharp transient events of skin color changes seen in RP. Chilblains, often referred to as pernio, manifests as inflammatory cutaneous lesions in patients exposed to non-freezing weather during late winter or early spring. These lesions typically present as painful erythrocyanotic discoloration often with cutaneous necrosis of the fingers or toes or both. It is frequently misdiagnosed as vasculitis or an embolic event [27].

Livedo reticularis is a violaceous, red or blue, reticular or mottled skin pattern with regular unbroken circles. Physiologic livedo reticularis, also known as cutis marmorata, mainly affects young women and most commonly occurs on the legs on exposure to cold, with gradual resolution on rewarming [28]. This can be seen during a cold response in patients with RP. Livedo racemosa is characterized by violaceous, red or blue, reticular or mottled skin pattern with irregular broken circles. It is seen in patients with vasculitis, vascular disease (e.g., secondary atheroemboli or thrombosis), or antiphospholipid syndrome [28].

Physical Examination

History provides the basis for priorities in clinical examination and subsequent management. After completing a thorough medical history, the clinician should have formulated a differential diagnosis to explain the patient's complaints. Physical examination is a critical tool to narrow down the differential diagnosis and guide further evaluation and management.

The physical examination for vascular disease should assess the cardiovascular system as a whole. Examination of the arterial system follows the pattern followed in other organ system examination. This includes inspection, palpation, and auscultation.

General Appearance

The patient's general appearance may provide initial clues for underlying vascular disease. Observations of patient's gait, body habitus, and vocalizations can provide important clues that will further guide the examination [12]. Special attention should be given to patients' vital signs. Blood pressure should be obtained from both arms. If a difference in blood pressure is noted, this must be accounted for (e.g., subclavian stenosis or aortic dissection)

Head and Neck Examination

Inspection may reveal the presence of xanthelasma or corneal arcus, which may suggest underlying hypercholesteremia. The presence of blue lips suggests central cyanosis. The presence of telangiectasia over the lips, tongue and buccal mucosa suggests presence of Osler–Weber–Rendu syndrome (also known as hereditary hemorrhagic telangiectasia). Iron deficiency anemia and pulmonary arteriovascular malformations are associated with this syndrome. The presence of facial plethora, neck distension (exacerbated by bending forward or lying down), and dilated chest veins should raise suspicion for superior vena cava syndrome.

Patients with Marfan syndrome (MFS) may have facial dolichocephaly (reduced cephalic index or head width:length ratio), enophthalmos, down-slanting palpebral fissures and retrognathia. Ehlers–Danlos syndrome is associated with acrogeria. This is defined by characteristic facial features such an emaciated face with prominent cheekbones and sunken cheeks. The eyes appear sunken or bulging, often with coloring around them and thin telangiectasia on the eyelids [29]. Loeys–Dietz syndrome is associated with arterial tortuosity with aortic aneurysms. Patients with this syndrome may have hypertelorism (widely spaced eyes), a split uvula or cleft palate, ectopia lentis and blue sclera [30]. Scleroderma may cause tightening of the skin in the face, with a characteristic beak-like face and paucity of wrinkles. Drawn pursed lips, shiny skin over the cheeks and forehead, and atrophy of muscles in the temple, face, and neck may also be seen with scleroderma.

Examination of the eye may also reveal clues for vascular diseases. Pallor of conjunctiva suggests presence of anemia. Ectopia lentis occurs in 50–80% with MFS [31]. It is detected on slit-lamp examination after maximal dilatation of the pupil and the lens is usually displaced upward and temporally. Fundoscopic examination is useful as a visualization of the arteriolar changes caused by hypertension (arteriovenous nicking, cotton wool patches, flame hemorrhages, papilledema), diabetes mellitus (neovascularization, microaneurysms), atherosclerosis (exudates, beading of the retinal artery), and atheromatous embolization (Hollenhorst plaques) [12].

The neck should be inspected for the presence of any abnormal pulsations and thyromegaly. On palpation, the carotid pulse should be carefully examined. The carotid pulse contour is very similar to that of the central aortic pulse. The onset of the ascending limb of the carotid pulse, compared with the central aortic pulse is delayed by only about 20 msec. For this reason examination of the carotid pulse provides the most accurate representation of changes in the central aortic pulse. The carotid arterial pulses are usually examined with the patient supine and the trunk of the patient's body slightly elevated. The fingers should be positioned between the larynx and the anterior border of the sternocleidomastoid muscle at the level of the cricoid cartilage. In palpating the pulse, the degree of pressure applied to the artery should be varied until the maximum pulsation is appreciated [32]. The clinician should note the volume and contour, as these can help to identify changes in left ventricular stroke volume and ejection velocity. When temporal arteritis is suspected, the temporal artery, located just anterior to the tragus of the ear, should be palpated. The strength of the pulse should be assessed, and the artery should be examined for thickening or dilatation, which may be signs of inflammation.

Auscultation of the carotid artery. The examination for carotid artery bruits should begin as high in the neck as possible, getting up under the mandible then slowly progressing down the course of the common carotid artery to the base of the neck. It is important to keep in mind that bruit alone is a poor predictor of either underlying carotid stenosis or stroke risk in asymptomatic patients. In a meta-analysis of symptomatic and asymptomatic patients, the sensitivity and specificity of a carotid bruit for a hemodynamically significant (70–99% stenosis) carotid lesion were 53% and 83%, respectively [33].

The proportion of patients with asymptomatic bruits who go on to have a stroke is low; the annual incidence of stroke ipsilateral to a bruit is 1–3% [34]. To differentiate carotid bruits from radiating cardiac murmurs, the examiner may move the stethoscope down the carotid; cardiac murmurs should increase in intensity as the stethoscope approaches the precordium. Moreover, a radiating cardiac murmurs will typically radiate to both carotids and a corresponding cardiac murmur will always be evident on precordial examination. Bruits originating from the subclavian artery are best detected in the supraclavicular fossa.

Vertebral artery bruits are best appreciated in the area posterior to the sterno-cleidomastoid muscles.

Chest

The patient should lie comfortably in the supine position with the trunk elevated 30–45°. The chest should be inspected for any deformities, abnormal pulsations, and dilated veins. Pectus carinatum (anterior displacement of sternum) and pectus excavatum are both observed in patients with MFS. The former, however, is believed to be more specific [35]. Thoracic aortic aneurysms can cause prominent pulsations in supraclavicular fossae and the suprasternal notch. A subxiphoid pulsation may occur with descending aortic aneurysm. Moreover, the suprasternal notch should be palpated for the presence of pulsations, which may indicate thoracic aneurysm involving the ascending aorta or aortic arch.

Describing full precordial examination is beyond the scope of this chapter; however, in assessing patients with PAD, there are certain precordial findings which are relevant. The presence of diffuse apex beat suggests the presence of systolic dysfunction. The presence of irregularly irregular heartbeats suggests the presence of atrial fibrillation, which is a major cause of cardio-embolization. The presence of high-pitched decrescendo murmur, which begins with the second heart sound (S2), suggests the presence of aortic regurgitation, which can be secondary to annular dilatation and ascending thoracic aortic aneurysm.

Abdominal Examination

The abdomen should be inspected for visible pulsations. Dilated veins may indicate vena caval obstructions or liver cirrhosis with portal hypertension.

Prominent pulsations may be associated with dilated or aneurysmal vessels, such as the descending aorta or iliac arteries. To palpate for abdominal aortic aneurysm, deep gentle palpation of the abdominal aorta should be performed using the fingers of both hands. The patient's abdominal muscles should be completely relaxed; such relaxation can be encouraged by asking the patient to flex the hips and by providing a pillow to support the head. It is important to note that palpation of the abdomen to detect AAA is safe and has never been reported to precipitate aortic rupture [36].

It is recommended that abdominal auscultation should be performed before palpation, given that the latter may increase peristalsis and thus make it difficult to appreciate abdominal bruits. The areas over the aorta, both renal arteries and the iliac arteries should be examined carefully for bruits.

As the abdominal aorta is a large and central vessel, aortic bruits are low-pitched and non-radiating. In contrast, the smaller mesenteric and renal arteries will have bruits of higher pitch, yet only true renal vascular bruits will radiate laterally to the flanks. Murmurs auscultated over either of the lower abdominal quadrants suggest iliac artery disease [12].

Lower Extremity Examination

Inspection of the extremities provides many clues for underlying vascular disease. Patients with underlying arterial insufficiency typically have cool and pale skin. Nail thickening and skin atrophy of the foot are observed in such patients. Hair loss was previously thought to occur in PAD but is now thought to be a non-specific finding. Ischemic ulcers may develop and are painful (may be painless in diabetics) and develop over pressure areas, e.g., lateral malleolus, heel, fifth metatarsal base and metatarsal heads. Ulcer margin is typically regular and its base is necrotic with no granulation tissue. It is important to differentiate these from venous ulcers, which develop predominantly above the medial or lateral malleoli in relation to long and short saphenous vein pathology, respectively. Venous ulcers are painful in one-third of patients, and pain often improves with leg elevation. Ulcer margins are typically irregular and the base is pink with granulation tissue. Ischemic ulcers also need to be differentiated from neuropathic ulcers. Table 2.2 illustrates the differential diagnosis of leg ulcers.

Digit ischemia (toe, finger) is the most common presentation of Buerger's disease. The presence of ischemic ulcerations in the upper or lower extremity with accompanying ischemic pain or gangrene of the digits in young heavy smokers less than 40–45 years of age should raise suspicion for Buerger's disease. Furthermore, superficial thrombophlebitis develops in 40–60% of patients with Buerger's disease. It can occur very early in the disease, even before symptoms and signs of digit ischemia are observed [37]. It presents as

Table 2.2 Characteristics of common foot and leg ulcers.

Origin	Cause	Location	Pain	Appearance
Arterial	Peripheral artery disease or Buerger's disease	Toes, foot and ankle	Severe	Pale base, dry, regular (punched out) margins, necrotic base with no granulation tissue
Venous	Venous insufficiency	Gaiter area; most commonly over medial malleolus	Mild	Irregular, moist and granulation tissue present
Neuropathic	Neuropathy, e.g., from diabetes	Foot/plantar surface, metatarsal heads and heel	None	Thick callus, well-defined wound margins with or without undermining Granulation tissue frequently present

erythema along the course of a vein, associated with a tender, cord-like vein on palpation. This superficial thrombophlebitis may be migratory and recurrent. Migrating thrombophlebitis (phlebitis saltans) in young heavy smokers is therefore highly suggestive of Buerger's disease. Deep vein thrombophlebitis is unusual in Buerger's disease and suggestive of an alternative diagnosis, such as Behçet's disease [37]. The presence of non-blanchable macular and papular lesions suggests the presence of cutaneous vasculitis.

Palpating for Pulses

The patient should be examined in a warm room with arrangements made so that the pulses can easily be examined from both sides of the bed. Palpation should be done using the fingertips and the intensity of the pulse graded as 0 (absent), 1 (diminished), or 2 (normal) [2].

The brachial artery is palpated in the antecubital fossa medial to the biceps tendon. With the elbow slightly flexed and externally rotated, the examiner's hand is then curled over the anterior aspect of the elbow to palpate the artery just medial to the biceps tendon.

The radial artery is palpated by curling the fingers around the distal radius, with the tips of the first, second, and third fingers aligned over the course of the artery [13]. The Allen test is used to verify patency of the radial, ulnar, palmar arch, and digital arteries. Allen test is a simple qualitative test that is used for this purpose. The patient is instructed to clench the fist. The examiner then compresses the radial and ulnar arteries simultaneously, and the patient is asked to relax the hand. The ulnar artery is then released and the time needed for maximal palmar blush to return is recorded. Return of the palmar blush within 5–10 seconds is considered normal[38]. In the reverse Allen test, the patient is instructed to clench the fist, both arteries are compressed, and the radial artery is released after the fingers are extended. Failure of palmar blush to return indicates occlusion of the radial artery or incomplete palmar arch.

The femoral artery emerges from beneath the inguinal ligament and is best palpated in mid inguinal point, which is half the distance between anterior superior iliac spine and symphysis pubis. It is palpated with the examiner standing on the ipsilateral side and the fingertips of the examining hand pressed firmly along the course the artery [13]. The sciatic artery is the earliest axial artery of the lower extremity in the human embryo, but it involutes in favor of the paired femoral arteries (superficial femoral artery and profunda femoris) [39]. Remnants of sciatic artery normally persist as popliteal and peroneal arteries. Failure of the sciatic artery to regress may result in femoral arterial hypoplasia, and therefore becoming the dominant inflow to the lower extremity [40]. Persistent sciatic arteries are prone to early atherosclerotic degeneration and aneurysm formation in up to 44% of cases. These aneurysms are characteristically located caudal to the sciatic notch [39].

The popliteal artery passes vertically through the deep portion of the popliteal space just lateral to the mid-plane. Generally this pulse is felt most conveniently with the patient in the supine position and the examiner's hands encircling and supporting the knee from each side. The pulse is detected by pressing deeply into the popliteal space with the supporting fingertips. As complete relaxation of the muscles is essential to this examination, the patient should be instructed to let the leg "go limp" and to allow the examiner to provide all the support needed [13]. A popliteal artery aneurysm (PAA) is suspected if a pulsatile popliteal mass is palpated at or above the level of the knee joint. PAA is defined when focal arterial dilation is identified and the diameter of the vessel is increased more than 50% relative to the vessel's normal diameter [41]. More than 50% are bilateral, and 33% of those with a PAA have a coexistent aortic aneurysm [42]. PAA is associated with increased risk of acute limb ischemia secondary to acute vessel thrombosis, distal embolization, and rupture, and thus early identification is critical.

The posterior tibial artery lies just posterior to the medial malleolus. It can be felt most readily by curling the fingers of the examining hand anteriorly around the ankle, indenting the soft tissues in the space between the medial malleolus and the Achilles tendon, above the calcaneus.

The thumb is applied to the opposite side of the ankle in a grasping fashion to provide stability. The dorsalis pedis artery is examined with the patient in the recumbent position and the ankle relaxed. The examiner stands at the foot of the examining table and places the fingertips transversely across the dorsum of the forefoot near the ankle. The artery usually lies near the center of the long axis of the foot, lateral to the extensor hallucis tendon, but it may be aberrant in location and often requires some searching. The dorsalis pedis pulse is congenitally absent in approximately 10% of individuals [32].

Different maneuvers have been described to assess for arterial insufficiency. The capillary refill test is performed by applying firm digital pressure to the plantar skin of the distal toe for 5 seconds. Transient pallor is considered normal, while a delay of greater than 5 seconds before return to usual skin color is considered as delayed refill. In the Buerger's test the patient lies supine and the leg is raised 45° and held passively for 2–3 minutes. In patients with PAD the toes and foot turn pale and there is emptying of veins over the dorsal foot. "Venous guttering" can also be observed. In step 2 of the Buerger's test, the patient is asked to sit on side of the bed with the legs dangling down. In patients with PAD, with dependency, the foot turns from pale to a deep red (brick red) color secondary to reactive hyperemia.

When thoracic outlet syndrome is suspected, thoracic outlet maneuvers should be done to assess the arterial flow patterns of the proximal vasculature. For the hyperabduction maneuver to assess for subclavian artery compression, the patient sits upright with the head looking forward. The examiner braces the patient's shoulder with one hand as the other hand continuously palpates the radial pulse while abducting and externally rotating the patient's arm. Alternatively, the examiner may use the first hand to auscultate the supraclavicular area for development of a subclavian artery bruit during the same maneuver. If the pulse is not diminished, a bruit is not induced, or symptoms are not produced in this position, the patient should then be asked to look to both the ipsilateral followed by the contralateral side with the chin extended (Adson's maneuver) [7]. If the test is still negative, the patient's arm or neck should be passively moved and the pulse amplitude assessed to evaluate for positional compression of the axillary or subclavian arteries on the affected side.

Finally, the costoclavicular maneuver evaluates for compression of the neurovascular bundle between the clavicle and first rib by having the patient stand at exaggerated military attention with the shoulders thrust backward and downward. Because many asymptomatic patients can have positive results, interpretation of all these tests must be made cautiously [12].

In one study, provocative tests have mean sensitivity and specificity values of 72% and 53%, respectively, with better values for the Adson test (positive predictive value [PPV], 85%) and the hyperabduction test (PPV, 92%) [43].

Auscultation

After palpating the artery, auscultation for a bruit should be performed. Bruits are detected by auscultation over the large and medium-sized arteries (e.g., carotid, brachial, abdominal aorta, femoral) with the diaphragm of the stethoscope using light to moderate pressure. Excessive pressure may produce, intensify, or prevent a bruit from being detected by indenting the vessel wall or occluding blood flow in the artery [32]. The subclavian artery is best auscultated in the ipsilateral supraclavicular fossa, while the femoral artery should be auscultated in the inguinal region and over Hunter's canal. The renal artery can be auscultated posteriorly just below the 12th rib.

The carotid bruit is of moderate value for detecting clinically relevant carotid stenosis. In a large meta-analysis, for detection of clinically relevant stenosis (>70%), carotid bruits had a pooled sensitivity of 0.53 (95% confidence interval [CI]: 0.5–0.55) and specificity 0.83 (95% CI: 0.82–0.84) [33].

The presence of common femoral artery bruit in asymptomatic patients is a moderately good predictor of PAD (likelihood ratio [LR] = 4.80; 95% CI: 2.40–9.50). The absence of a bruit, however, doesn't exclude disease (LR = 0.83; 95% CI: 0.73–0.95) [44, 45]. The examiner should always auscultate over hunter's canal for bruits of superficial femoral artery. A bruit detected in the inguinal region can have several sources, and different techniques can aid in localizing the source. First, the examiner should listen both proximal and distal to the area where the bruit is first auscultated. An iliac artery bruit decreases in intensity as the auscultation moves distally into the femoral region. If, on the other hand, a bruit is louder in the femoral area and softer in the iliac fossa, it is likely secondary to disease of the common femoral artery, the superficial femoral artery and/or the profunda femoral artery [12]. The bruit occlusion test can also be used to localize the source of the bruit. This test is performed by compressing the superficial femoral artery near the apex of the femoral triangle. If the bruit disappears or decreases in intensity, a stenosis is more likely to be present in the common or superficial femoral artery. A bruit caused by a lesion in the profunda femoral artery will instead become louder with compression [12].

References

1 Eraso LH, Fukaya E, Mohler ER *et al.* Peripheral arterial disease, prevalence and cumulative risk factor profile analysis. Eur J Prev Cardiol. 2014; 21: 704–11.

2 Norgren L, Hiatt WR, Dormandy JA, *et al.* Inter-Society Consensus for the Management of Peripheral Arterial Disease (TASC II). J Vasc Surg. 2007; 45: S5-67.

3 Kullo IJ, Bailey KR, Kardia SLR, *et al.* Ethnic differences in peripheral arterial disease in the NHLBI Genetic Epidemiology Network of Arteriopathy (GENOA) study. Vasc Med Lond Engl. 2003; 8: 237–42.

4 Selvin E, Erlinger TP. Prevalence of and risk factors for peripheral arterial disease in the United States: results from the National Health and Nutrition Examination Survey, 1999–2000. Circulation. 2004; 110: 738–43.

5 Agarwal S. The association of active and passive smoking with peripheral arterial disease: results from NHANES 1999–2004. Angiology. 2009; 60: 335–45.

6 Fowkes FG, Housley E, Cawood EH, *et al.* Edinburgh Artery Study: prevalence of asymptomatic and symptomatic peripheral arterial disease in the general population. Int J Epidemiol. 1991; 20: 384–92.

7 Selvin E, Marinopoulos S, Berkenblit G, *et al.* Meta-analysis: glycosylated hemoglobin and cardiovascular disease in diabetes mellitus. Ann Intern Med. 2004; 141: 421–31.

8 Murabito JM, D'Agostino RB, Silbershatz H, Wilson WF. Intermittent claudication. A risk profile from The Framingham Heart Study. Circulation. 1997; 96: 44–9.

9 Heart Protection Study Collaborative Group. MRC/BHF Heart Protection Study of antioxidant vitamin supplementation in 20, 536 high-risk individuals: a randomised placebo-controlled trial. Lancet. 2002; 360: 23–33.

10 Easton JD, Saver JL, Albers GW, *et al.* Definition and evaluation of transient ischemic attack: a scientific statement for healthcare professionals from the American Heart Association/American Stroke Association Stroke Council;

Council on Cardiovascular Surgery and Anesthesia; Council on Cardiovascular Radiology and Intervention; Council on Cardiovascular Nursing; and the Interdisciplinary Council on Peripheral Vascular Disease. The American Academy of Neurology affirms the value of this statement as an educational tool for neurologists. Stroke J Cereb Circ. 2009; 40: 2276–93.

11 Tao W-D, Liu M, Fisher M, *et al*. Posterior versus anterior circulation infarction: how different are the neurological deficits? Stroke. 2012; 43: 2060–5.

12 Dieter RS, Dieter RA, Jr, Dieter RA, III. Peripheral Arterial Disease. New York: McGraw-Hill Medical, 2009.

13 Wilterdink JL, Easton JD. Vascular event rates in patients with atherosclerotic cerebrovascular disease. Arch Neurol. 1992; 49: 857–63.

14 Contorni L. [The vertebro-vertebral collateral circulation in obliteration of the subclavian artery at its origin]. Minerva Chir. 1960; 15: 268–71.

15 Dieter RS. The Dieter test. Expert Rev Cardiovasc Ther. 2009; 7: 221.

16 Levitt B, Richter JE. Dysphagia lusoria: a comprehensive review. Dis Esophagus Off J Int Soc Dis Esophagus ISDE. 2007; 20: 455–60.

17 Neri E, Toscano T, Papalia U, *et al*. Proximal aortic dissection with coronary malperfusion: presentation, management, and outcome. J Thorac Cardiovasc Surg. 2001; 121: 552–60.

18 Assar AN, Zarins CK. Ruptured abdominal aortic aneurysm: a surgical emergency with many clinical presentations. Postgrad Med. J. 2009; 85: 268–73.

19 Hellmann DB, Grand DJ, Freischlag JA. Inflammatory abdominal aortic aneurysm. JAMA. 2007; 297: 395–400.

20 Cheuk W, Chan JKC. IgG4-related sclerosing disease: a critical appraisal of an evolving clinicopathologic entity. Adv Anat Pathol. 2010; 17: 303–32.

21 Kasashima S, Zen Y, Kawashima A, *et al*. Inflammatory abdominal aortic aneurysm: close relationship to IgG4-related periaortitis. Am J Surg Pathol. 2008; 32: 197–204.

22 Moawad J, Gewertz BL. Chronic mesenteric ischemia. Clinical presentation and diagnosis. Surg Clin North Am. 1997; 77: 357–69.

23 Myers SA, Johanning JM, Stergiou N, *et al*. Claudication distances and the Walking Impairment Questionnaire best describe the ambulatory limitations in patients with symptomatic peripheral arterial disease. J Vasc Surg. 2008; 47: 550–5.

24 Coyne KS, Margolis MK, Gilchrist KA, *et al*. Evaluating effects of method of administration on Walking Impairment Questionnaire. J Vasc Surg. 2003; 38: 296–304.

25 Chikura B, Moore T, Manning J, *et al*. Thumb involvement in Raynaud's phenomenon as an indicator of underlying connective tissue disease. J Rheumatol. 2010; 37: 783–6.

26 Ablett CT, Hackett LA. Hypothenar hammer syndrome: case reports and brief review. Clin Med Res. 2008; 6: 3–8.

27 Prakash S, Weisman MH. Idiopathic chilblains. Am J Med. 2009; 122: 1152–5.

28 Uthman IW, Khamashta MA. Livedo racemosa: a striking dermatological sign for the antiphospholipid syndrome. J Rheumatol. 2006; 33: 2379–82.

29 Germain DP. Ehlers–Danlos syndrome type IV. Orphanet J Rare Dis. 2007; 2: 32.

30 Loeys BL, Schwarze U, Holm T *et al.* Aneurysm syndromes caused by mutations in the TGF-beta receptor. N Engl J Med. 2006; 355: 788–98.

31 Tsipouras P, Del Mastro R, Sarfarazi M *et al.* Genetic linkage of the Marfan syndrome, ectopia lentis, and congenital contractural arachnodactyly to the fibrillin genes on chromosomes 15 and 5. The International Marfan Syndrome Collaborative Study. N Engl J Med. 1992; 326: 905–9.

32 Walker HK, Hall WD, Hurst JW, eds. Clinical Methods: the History, Physical, and Laboratory Examinations, 3rd edn. Boston, MA: Butterworths, 1990.

33 McColgan P, Bentley P, McCarron M, Sharma P. Evaluation of the clinical utility of a carotid bruit. QJM Mon J Assoc Physicians. 2012; 105: 1171–7.

34 Chambers BR, Norris JW. Outcome in patients with asymptomatic neck bruits. N Engl J Med. 1986; 315: 860–5.

35 Loeys BL, Dietz HC, Braverman AC, *et al.* The revised Ghent nosology for the Marfan syndrome. J Med Genet. 2010; 47: 476–85.

36 Lederle FA, Simel DL. The rational clinical examination. Does this patient have abdominal aortic aneurysm? JAMA. 1999; 281: 77–82.

37 Vijayakumar A, Tiwari R, Kumar Prabhuswamy V. Thromboangiitis obliterans (Buerger's disease) – current practices. Int J Inflamm. 2013. Online: https://doi.org/10.1155/2013/156905.

38 Kotowycz MA, Dzavík V. Radial artery patency after transradial catheterization. Circ Cardiovasc Interv. 2012; 5: 127–33.

39 Sindel T, Yilmaz S, Onur R, Sindel M. Persistent sciatic artery. Radiologic features and patient management. Saudi Med J. 2006; 27: 721–4.

40 Wu H-Y, Yang Y-J, Lai C-H, *et al.* Bilateral persistent sciatic arteries complicated with acute left lower limb ischemia. J Formos Med Assoc Taiwan Yi Zhi. 2007; 106: 1038–42.

41 Johnston KW, Rutherford RB, Tilson MD, *et al.* Suggested standards for reporting on arterial aneurysms. Subcommittee on Reporting Standards for Arterial Aneurysms, Ad Hoc Committee on Reporting Standards, Society for Vascular Surgery and North American Chapter, International Society for Cardiovascular Surgery. J Vasc Surg. 1991; 13: 452–8.

42 Carpenter JP, Barker CF, Roberts B, *et al.* artery aneurysms: current management and outcome. J Vasc Surg. 1994; 19: 65–72 (discussion 72–3).

43 Gillard J, Pérez-Cousin M, Hachulla E *et al*. Diagnosing thoracic outlet syndrome: contribution of provocative tests, ultrasonography, electrophysiology, and helical computed tomography in 48 patients. Jt Bone Spine Rev Rhum. 2001; 68: 416–24.

44 Khan NA, Rahim SA, Anand SS, *et al*. Does the clinical examination predict lower extremity peripheral arterial disease? JAMA. 2006; 295: 536–46.

45 Walker KM, Messick BH, Kaufman L. Clinical inquiries: how should you evaluate an asymptomatic patient with a femoral or iliac artery bruit? J Fam Pract. 2009; 58: 217–8.

3

Vascular Laboratory Evaluation of Peripheral Artery Disease

Thomas Rooke

Mayo Clinic, Rochester, MN, USA

Introduction

The definition of peripheral artery disease (PAD) classically includes all forms of extracoronary and extracranial arterial pathologies, but in practice the term is usually reserved for atherosclerotic disease affecting the (primarily lower) extremities [1]. When PAD involves the legs it produces signs and symptoms like claudication, ischemic rest pain, or skin ulceration. If these problems are present (based on the patient's history, physical examination, or other clinical characteristics) the next step in the evaluation for possible PAD is often a non-invasive "vascular laboratory" assessment. Modern vascular laboratories use a variety of testing modalities (either alone or in combination) to obtain three general types of diagnostic information.

Anatomic

These studies (typically employing grayscale or other ultrasound imaging techniques) provide information about the physical appearance of blood vessels and can be used to address specific anatomical questions about the arteries. For example, are regions of stenosis/obstruction/occlusion present? If so, where are these lesions located? What is their gross appearance (are the lesions calcified, echolucent, etc.)? Are there other structural abnormalities such as aneurysm, dissection, and so on?

Hemodynamic

Certain modalities can assess abnormalities in blood flow at a particular location of interest. For example, if an arterial segment appears to be narrow (based on an imaging study), does it obstruct flow? Is there a Doppler velocity

Peripheral Artery Disease, Second Edition. Edited by Emile R. Mohler and Michael R. Jaff.
© 2017 John Wiley & Sons Ltd. Published 2017 by John Wiley & Sons Ltd.

gradient across a particular stenotic lesion (and therefore presumably a blood pressure gradient as well)? How hemodynamically "severe" is the obstruction associated with this gradient?

Functional

Some tests primarily assess the impact of arterial disease on the downstream organs and tissues. For example, if occlusive lesions are present (and appear to be sufficient to cause hemodynamically significant impairment of blood flow), does this obstruction also impair the function of the limb? Is the obstruction sufficient to explain signs or symptoms such as claudication, ischemic rest pain, or skin ulceration?

Although *physiological* testing (i.e., tests that assess *hemodynamic* or *functional* status) are sometimes thought of as being "less accurate" or "less valuable" than imaging studies (e.g., imaging obtained using ultrasound, magnetic resonance [MR], computed tomography [CT], or even direct angiography) the information provided typically compliments anatomical testing and allows the practitioner to gain a fuller understanding of a patient's arterial pathology.

Physiological Testing

Background/History

Physiological Invasive Testing

In 1733 the Reverend Steven Hales connected a 9-foot-long glass tube to the "left crural artery" of a mare and determined the animal's systolic blood pressure by observing the height to which the column of blood rose. Work by Poiseuille and (later) Ludwig in the 1800s refined and simplified the approach to direct (invasive) arterial pressure measurement, and the first (direct) measurement of human blood pressure occurred in 1856 [2]. During the 1940s, direct measurement of arterial blood pressure became a routine clinical practice [3]. Unfortunately, direct blood pressure measurement (employing arterial cannulation with tubes, catheterization with needles, etc.) has limited clinical utility owing to the difficulty, time, inconvenience, and pain associated with the procedures. Before limb arterial blood pressure measurement would become widespread in its application, less invasive methods were needed.

Physiological Non-Invasive Testing

By the end of the 1700s, physician-scientists like Riva-Rocci and Korotkoff were developing non-invasive methods for measuring arterial blood pressure in limbs [2]. The introduction of strain gauges enabled clinicians to detect and record arterial pulsations, and by combining strain-gauge *plethysmography* with *sphygmomanometry* (using pneumatic arterial occlusion cuffs placed around the limb) it became possible to measure arterial pressure at various levels of the extremity. In the 1950s, Winsor [4] demonstrated that blood pressure could be determined with this approach (and that it was reduced in limbs with PAD), and in 1970 Yao [5] showed that reductions in limb blood pressure measurements (especially when compared with "central" arterial blood pressure) correlated with the severity of PAD. At roughly this same time, Carter demonstrated the value of exercise as a means to "unmask" (or assess the impact of) milder forms of PAD [6]. Satomura's development of the ultrasonic Doppler in the 1950s added another tool that would eventually enter routine use in the vascular laboratory [7].

Vascular Laboratory

The first non-invasive vascular laboratory was established at Massachusetts General Hospital in the 1940s [8], and during the 1950s and 1960s clinically focused vascular laboratories began to appear in the United States and elsewhere [9]. The vascular laboratory at Roper Hospital in Charleston, South Carolina, was founded in 1956 and is the oldest vascular laboratory in continuous operation in the United States [10].

Doppler

Doppler devices detect the frequency shift that occurs when ultrasound waves encounter moving blood; the result can be viewed as a physical printout or heard as an audio signal. Although the physics behind the various Doppler modalities in current use (continuous wave, pulsed wave, color flow, etc.) are beyond the scope of this work, their application in the vascular laboratory is relatively simple. Basically, Doppler devices are used clinically in two major ways: motion detection and waveform analysis.

Motion Detection

Because Doppler accurately detects the motion of blood, it can be used in conjunction with arterial occlusion pneumatic cuffs to determine the blood pressure at a given limb level. To do this a cuff is wrapped around the limb and inflated to a pressure sufficient to occlude arterial flow. The Doppler probe is placed over the artery distal to the cuff, and as the air in the cuff is slowly released, the pressure at which flow in the artery resumes is identified. This value represents the (systolic) arterial pressure at the level of the air cuff. By moving the cuff along the limb (or employing multiple cuffs placed at various levels) and repeating the process, pressures can be obtained at virtually any level of the limb. Arterial blockages caused by PAD or other problems can be identified and localized when a drop-off in pressure, a pressure gradient, is detected in the limb.

Waveform Analysis

The arterial Doppler signal can be analyzed for components related to its contour and shape. The normal arterial Doppler signal is triphasic and demonstrates forward flow during systole, reverse flow during early diastole, and a return of forward flow during late diastole (Figure 3.1a). When obstruction to arterial flow occurs proximal to the site of interrogation, the downstream waveform changes in predictable ways; the amplitude of the wave is dampened, early forward flow is delayed, flow reversal is delayed or lost, and late diastole forward flow is lost (Figure 3.1b). The waveform takes on a monophasic shape. By interrogating the artery at multiple levels, the presence and location of occlusive lesions can be identified in the limb.

Plethysmography

During the 1950s and 1960s, strain gauges made of mercury-in-rubber or silastic became available for clinical use; air-filled plethysmographic cuffs were introduced later and have largely replaced strain gauges in most commercial devices. Regardless of the mechanism, the technique of plethysmography for the study of arteries has become relatively standardized. To perform a test the device is wrapped around the limb or digit at a point of interest (Figure 3.2). With each cardiac pulsation the underlying artery(ies) (and therefore, the limb) expands transiently as a bolus of arterial blood passes through and distends the

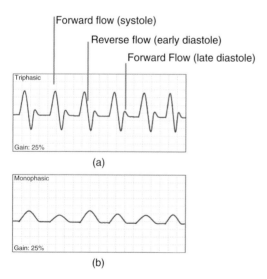

Figure 3.1 (a) Normal Doppler signal showing triphasic flow. (b) Monophasic Doppler signal obtained distal to a hemodynamically significant arterial lesion. The wave is dampened and delayed. Note the absence of forward flow in late diastole.

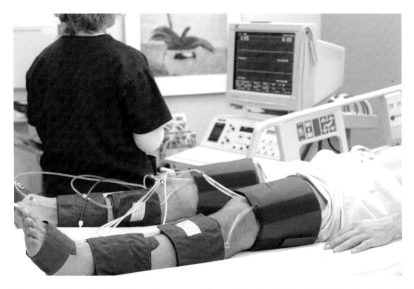

Figure 3.2 A series of pulse-volume recording cuffs placed at multiple levels of the limb(s).

vessel(s). Limb expansion displaces air from the cuff, creating changes in volume and pressure that can be recorded.

Like Doppler, plethysmography can be used to assess arterial patency in two major ways. In its simplest form plethysmography is a method for *pulse detection*; by placing the device distal to a pneumatic occlusion cuff, a plethysmograph can be used in lieu of a Doppler to measure limb arterial blood pressure at any level of interest. Plethysmography, like Doppler, can also be used to assess the *waveform* of arterial pulsations. This approach, most often called "pulse volume recording" (PVR), likewise examines features of the underlying pulse wave such as "amplitude" and "contour" to determine the presence of PAD [11], and just as the Doppler signal can be obtained and analyzed at any level of the limb, so can the PVR. Although the Doppler and PVR might seem to provide similar information about arterial pulsations, the PVR tends to be easier to apply, simpler to use, and more reproducible than the Doppler for routine clinical practice.

PVR Amplitude
The height of the arterial wave detected by PVR is relatively reproducible as long as characteristics such as cuff volume and pressure are carefully controlled; even factors like the presence or absence of edema have surprisingly little effect on amplitude [12]. In contrast, changes in physiological variables such as vasoconstriction/vasodilation will dramatically influence pulse amplitude.

PVR Contour

The PVR waveform (Figure 3.3) is dependent upon the limb level from which it is obtained, owing to changes produced by wave attenuation, elasticity of the artery, wave reflection, and other factors. The presence of PAD proximal to the site of PVR measurement will affect wave contour in a variety of ways: attenuation of the initial rate of rise, delay in the pulse peak, delayed rate of fall in the passing wave, and absence of a reflected diastolic pulse wave. These changes become more noticeable and dramatic as the severity of PAD worsens.

By employing air cuffs to occlude venous outflow from the limb, plethysmography can also be used to measure *arterial flow* into the limb. Venous (*outflow*) occlusion causes arterial blood (*inflow*) entering the limb to become "trapped." As blood entering the limb through the arteries is trapped, the volume of the limb increases. The rate of increase in limb volume can be measured by plethysmography and corresponds to the magnitude of arterial inflow [13]. A blunted waveform indicates a more proximal obstructive lesion. Although the measurement of resting arterial flow has minimal clinical utility in most settings (and is therefore not routinely performed by most vascular laboratories), there are occasions where it may be useful (e.g., in response to certain provocative maneuvers such as the administration of a vasodilator).

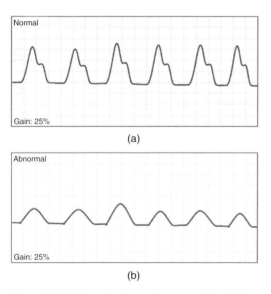

(a)

(b)

Figure 3.3 (a) Normal pulse-volume recording (PVR) waveform. The "notch" in the downslope (dicrotic notch) results from the reflected pulse wave during diastole. (b) PVR obtained distal to a hemodynamically significant arterial lesion. The amplitude is reduced and the contour has changed.

Ankle–Brachial Index (ABI) and Segmental Pressures

The non-invasive measurement of lower extremity arterial pressure – particularly at the ankle – has evolved as the most useful and popular test for PAD [14]. The classic ABI is a pressure index obtained by measuring the systolic blood pressure at the ankle using an arterial occlusion cuff placed over the lower calf, and a hand-held continuous-wave Doppler [15]. Pressures are obtained from both the dorsalis pedis and the posterior tibial arteries; the higher of these values is used for further calculations (Figure 3.4). Systolic brachial blood pressure is also measured in both arms and the higher of the values is used for further calculations. The ABI is subsequently determined by

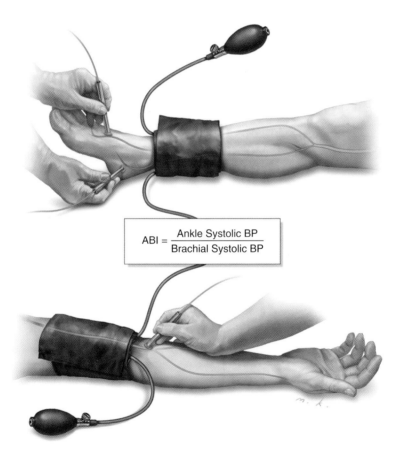

$$ABI = \frac{\text{Ankle Systolic BP}}{\text{Brachial Systolic BP}}$$

Figure 3.4 The ankle–brachial pressure index (ABI) for a limb is obtained by dividing the ankle pressure (using the higher of the dorsalis pedis or posterior tibial pressure) by the arm pressure (the higher obtained from either arm).

dividing the higher systolic ankle pressure by the highest brachial pressure in either arm. In recent years, devices have been developed which can use a variety of pulse-sensing technologies such as laser Doppler [16], plethysmography, or oscillometry (coupled with automated inflatable cuffs) to determine ABIs; these devices can simplify and speed the measurement of ABI and may be accurate enough for routine clinical use [17]. Numerous studies have shown that the ABI not only accurately predicts the presence and severity of PAD, but also correlates with the presence of atherosclerosis elsewhere (and therefore predicts coronary artery disease, cardiac events, mortality, and other significant outcomes).

The "normal" value for ABI is defined as 1.00–1.40 (systolic pressure in the leg is typically higher than arm pressure, owing to the amplification of the pulse wave as it moves distally from the heart). Values ≤ 0.90 are "abnormal" and suggest the presence of PAD or other forms of arterial obstruction. Values in the range 0.91–0.99 are considered "borderline" for the diagnosis of arterial obstruction [18]. When ABI > 1.40 is obtained, the most likely explanation is that the medial layer of the artery is calcified, rigid, and no longer compressible by the occlusion sphygmomanometer. This is typically seen in patients with long-standing diabetes, advanced stage, and certain other conditions. There is evidence suggesting that the cardiovascular risk associated with non-compressible arteries may be increased [19]; when necessary, additional information regarding arterial patency can often be obtained by measuring the pressure in the great toe (i.e., the toe–brachial index) [20]. The presence of underlying intimal layer atherosclerosis is common (more than 60% by one report) in the setting of a supernormal pressure in the leg [21]. Even when calcification affects the vessels of the calf and ankle, the toe arteries usually remain compressible. Although toe pressures are often less reproducible than those from the ankle, they can still provide important diagnostic information.

Exercise [22] may be used to identify PAD in situations where the disease is mild and does not cause a reduction in ABI at rest (Figure 3.5). During exercise (which is most often treadmill walking) the systemic (brachial) blood pressure and lower extremity (ankle) pressures normally rise in tandem. When hemodynamically significant PAD is present, the arm pressure rises with exercise as predicted, but the limb pressure response is diminished. In some cases ankle pressure may fall despite a rise in arm pressure; this produces a marked decrease in the ABI. Disease severity is reflected by the walking distance, the development of exercise-induced symptoms, the decrease in blood pressure during/after exercise, the post-exercise blood pressure recovery time (blood pressure typically takes up to 5–10 minutes or more to recover following exercise depending upon disease severity, but may take longer when disease is severe) and other changes. In some laboratories, electrocardiographic monitoring is

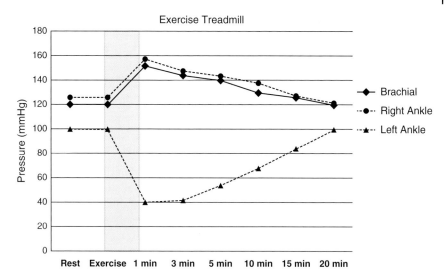

Figure 3.5 Exercise study in patient with left lower limb peripheral artery disease (PAD). In normal limbs (right), both the arm and leg pressure rise with exercise. In limbs with PAD (left) the arm pressure rises but the ankle pressure falls. The exercise capacity, post-exercise pressure fall, and pressure recovery time reflect the severity of the PAD.

performed during exercise; this enables the exercise test to serve as a screen for occult coronary artery disease.

There is no universally agreed upon protocol for exercise testing in the vascular laboratory [23]. Many laboratories use a "fixed" protocol involving exercise for a predetermined maximum time or distance, a standard speed, and a predetermined gradient (e.g., a maximum of 5 minutes of walking at 2 mph up a gradient of 10°). Other laboratories utilize protocols that involve progressive increases in exercise intensity (e.g., a progressive increase in speed and gradient to determine the maximal performance possible). In situations where ambulation is not feasible, protocols involving dobutamine infusion [24] or toe-tip exercise [25] may be substitutes for walking protocols.

Tissue Perfusion

Techniques for assessing skin blood flow have been commercially developed and are used in many vascular laboratories. Early devices for this purpose include the *photoplethysmograph* (PPG) [26]; although these devices are still in wide use the information they provide is largely qualitative and difficult to quantify. Newer approaches often use laser Doppler probes to assess microvascular skin perfusion. Laser Doppler technology, while more objective than PPG, also has limitations with quantification and interpretation. Like PVR, laser Doppler can be used to assess cutaneous (small vessel) wave amplitude and contour, or it can be coupled with pneumatic cuffs to determine the pressure (applied to the probe) at which the underlying skin blood flow ceases (this value represents the skin perfusion pressure). These devices are useful for assessing disease severity and predicting the potential for ulcers to heal, especially in patients with diabetes or other conditions that affect small cutaneous blood vessels [27–29].

Transcutaneous Oximetry (TcPO$_2$)

An alternative method for assessing the adequacy of skin perfusion is to measure TcPO$_2$ [30]. This test uses Clark-type oxygen sensing electrodes that are attached to the skin (with air-tight seals) and allowed to equilibrate (Figure 3.6). Oxygen diffuses out of the skin, and the subsequent steady-state oxygen tension correlates with the adequacy of skin blood flow; this can be used to diagnose or assess limb ischemia, predict wound or amputation site healing, among other things [31]. Depending upon the equipment used and the protocol employed, TcPO$_2$ values greater than 30–40 mmHg are predictive of wound healing. Factors such as venous disease, cutaneous edema, inflammation, and others can influence the measurement of TcPO$_2$ and complicate the interpretation of findings.

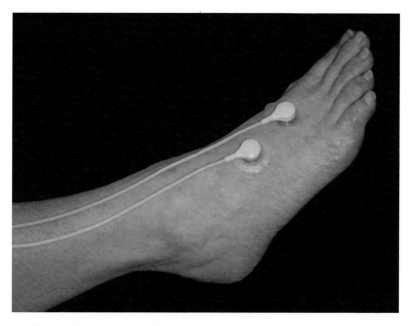

Figure 3.6 Transcutaneous oximetry electrodes are placed over points of interest and sealed to the skin with air-tight tape.

Duplex Scanning

Background/History

In 1974 Strandness introduced ultrasonic duplex scanning into clinical practice [32, 33]. His device combined two-dimensional (2D) grayscale ultrasound imaging with Doppler velocity measurements, and for the first time anatomic and hemodynamic information could be obtained non-invasively from almost any artery in the body [34]. The technique has been aggressively and steadily refined since its inception, and the availability of duplex scanning has proliferated as its popularity has grown. Duplex scanning is now so widely available that it is found in virtually every vascular laboratory; indeed, in most laboratories, it is the main (and sometimes only) technology used for arterial assessment. For certain arteries (such as the carotid or abdominal aorta) it is typically the only non-invasive method for assessing PAD in the outpatient setting. In some practices, duplex scanning has reduced or even eliminated the need for angiography (including MR, CT, or conventional angiography).

Imaging (Anatomy)

B-mode imaging refers to an ultrasonic approach that creates a 2D image plane allowing the operator to "slice" through the area of interest. These images (which are dynamic and obtained in real time) provide anatomic and structural information that may be critical for identifying or understanding arterial pathology (Figure 3.7). For example, imaging can identify and localize areas of arterial narrowing, aneurysms (both true and false), extrinsic arterial compression, calcifications, graft abnormalities such as kinking, and numerous other arterial abnormalities. Ultrasound imaging has shown impressive utility as a

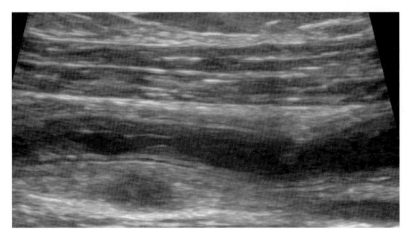

Figure 3.7 Grayscale image of femoral artery. Note the irregular lumen with areas of narrowing.

means for assessing plaque morphology in patients with PAD, although plaque characteristics are not commonly described in vascular laboratory reports due to issues regarding inter-observer variability. Over the past decade the potential for ultrasound imaging to assess the carotid intimal medial thickness (IMT) – a potential risk factor for the development of PAD – has become an area of intense research interest [35].

Doppler (Hemodynamic)

Combining a pulsed-wave Doppler with 2D imaging (duplex scanning) enables the operator to measure blood flow velocity at precise locations within the artery. Areas of anatomic arterial narrowing can be interrogated with the Doppler component to determine whether there is hemodynamic significance to the lesion, and based upon well-studied velocity criteria many lesions can be categorized according to severity. Technical advances have allowed modern duplex scanners to use color scales to indicate blood flow velocity; this has led to the highly popular "color flow" scans that can be performed with most equipment (Figure 3.8). Improvement in duplex technology continues to evolve on a steady basis.

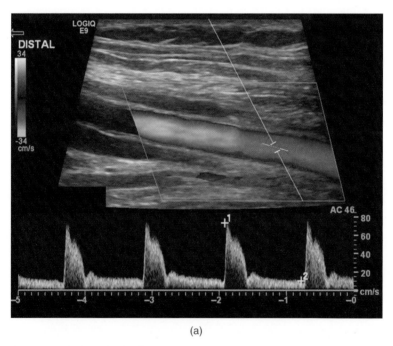

(a)

Figure 3.8 (a) Normal color flow duplex scan. The peak pulse-wave Doppler velocities are between 60 and 80 cm/s. (b) Color flow duplex scan of stenotic artery. The peak pulsed-wave velocities across the stenotic lesion are greater than 400 cm/s.

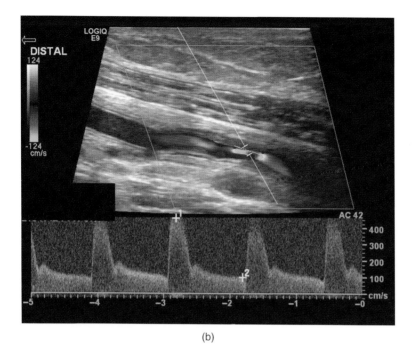

(b)

Figure 3.8 (*Continued*)

Vascular Laboratory Accreditation

More than 20 years ago the Intersocietal Accreditation Commission (IAC) began a program of voluntary vascular laboratory accreditation [36]; other groups have subsequently developed competing programs for laboratory accreditation. Laboratories accredited by the IAC or other organizations must meet specific standards designed to ensure the performance of safe, quality, non-invasive studies. Accreditation has helped to ensure the continued improvement in vascular laboratories in the United States and around the world.

References

1 Criqui MH, Fronek A, Barrett-Connor E, *et al.* The prevalence of peripheral arterial disease in a defined population. Circulation. 1985; 71(3): 510–5.
2 Booth J. A short history of blood pressure measurement. Proc R Soc Med. 1977; 70: 793–9.
3 Peterson LH, Dripps RD, Risman GC. A method for recording the arterial pressure pulse and blood pressure in man. Am Heart J. 1949; 37(5): 771–82.

4 Winsor T. Influence of arterial disease on the systolic blood pressure gradients of the extremity. Am J Med Sci. 1950; 220: 117.

5 Yao ST. Haemodynamic studies in peripheral arterial disease. Br J Surg. 1970; 57: 761–6.

6 Carter SA. Response of ankle systolic pressure to leg exercise in mild or questionable arterial disease. N Engl J Med. 1972; 287(12): 578–2.

7 Satomura S. Ultrasonic Doppler method for the inspection of cardiac function. J Acoust Soc Am. 1957; 29(11): 1181–5.

8 Division of Vascular and Endovascular Surgery, Massachusetts General Hospital. http://www.massgeneral.org/surgery/services/procedure. aspx?id=2292. Accessed: March 2017.

9 Harris JP. Early development of the vascular laboratory in Australia. ANZ J Surg. 2003; 73: 540–3.

10 Medical Society of South Carolina. http://www.medsocietysc.com/history/. Accessed: March 2017.

11 Darling RC, Raines JK, Brener BJ, Austen WG. Quantitative segmental pulse volume recorder: a clinical tool. Surgery. 1972; 72(6): 873–7.

12 Lewis JE, Owens DR. The pulse volume recorder as a measure of peripheral vascular status in people with diabetes mellitus. Diabetes Technol Ther. 2010; 12(1): 75–80.

13 Wilkinson IB, Webb DJ. Venous occlusion plethysmography in cardiovascular research: methodology and clinical applications. Br J Clin Pharmacol. 2001; 52(6): 631–46.

14 Xu D, Zou L, Xing Y, *et al.* Diagnostic value of ankle-brachial index in peripheral arterial disease: a meta-analysis. Can J Cardiol. 2013; 29(4): 492–8.

15 Aboyans V, Criqui MH, Abraham P, *et al.* Measurement and interpretation of the ankle-brachial index: a scientific statement from the American Heart Association. Circulation. 2012; 126: 2890–909.

16 Ludyga T, Kuczmik WB, Kazibudzki M, *et al.* Ankle-brachial pressure index estimated by laser Doppler in patients suffering from peripheral arterial obstructive disease. Ann Vasc Surg. 2007; 21(4): 452–7.

17 Hoyer C, Sandermann J, Petersen LJ. Randomised diagnostic accuracy study of a fully automated portable device for diagnosing peripheral arterial disease by measuring the toe-brachial index. Eur J Vasc Endovasc Surg. 2013; 45(1): 57–64.

18 Rooke T, Hirsch A, Misra S, *et al.* ACCF/AHA focused update of the guideline for the management of patients with peripheral artery disease (updating the 2005 guideline): a report of the American College of Cardiology Foundation/ American Heart Association Task Force on Practice Guidelines. Circulation. 2011; 124: 2020–45.

19 Criqui MH, McClelland RL, McDermott MM, *et al.* The ankle-brachial index and incident cardiovascular events in the MESA (Multi-Ethnic Study of Atherosclerosis). J Am Coll Cardiol. 2010; 56: 1506–12.

20 Hoyer C, Sandermann J, Petersen LJ. The toe-brachial index in the diagnosis of peripheral arterial disease. J Vasc Surg. 2013; 58(1): 231–8.

21 Suominen V, Rantanen T, Venermo M, *et al*. Prevalence and risk factors of PAD among patients with elevated ABI. Eur J Vasc Endovasc Surg. 2008; 35: 709–14.

22 Stein R, Hriljac I, Halperin JL, *et al*. Limitation of the resting ankle-brachial index in symptomatic patients with peripheral arterial disease. Vasc Med. 2006; 11(1): 29–33.

23 Riebe D, Patterson RB, Braun CM. Comparison of two progressive treadmill tests in patients with peripheral arterial disease. Vasc Med. 2001; 6: 215.

24 Wysokinski WE, Spittell PC, Pellikka PA, *et al*. Dobutamine effect on ankle-brachial pressure index in patients with peripheral arterial occlusive disease. New noninvasive test for evaluation of peripheral circulation? Int Angiol. 1998; 17(3): 201–7.

25 McPhail IR, Spittell PC, Weston SA, Bailey KR. Intermittent claudication: an objective office-based assessment. J Am Coll Cardiol. 2001; 37(5): 1381–5.

26 Parameswaran GI, Brand K, Dolan J. Pulse oximetry as a potential screening tool for lower extremity arterial disease in asymptomatic patients with diabetes mellitus. Arch Intern Med. 2005; 165(4): 442–6.

27 Castronuovo JJ Jr, Adera HM, Smiell JM, Price RM. Skin perfusion pressure measurement is valuable in the diagnosis of critical limb ischemia. J Vasc Surg. 1997; 26(4): 629–37.

28 Tsai FW, Tulsyan N, Jones DN, *et al*. Skin perfusion pressure of the foot is a good substitute for toe pressure in the assessment of limb ischemia. J Vasc Surg. 2000; 32(1): 32–6.

29 Yamada T, Ohta T, Ishibashi H, *et al*. Clinical reliability and utility of skin perfusion pressure measurement in ischemic limbs – comparison with other noninvasive diagnostic methods. J Vasc Surg. 2008; 47(2): 318–23.

30 Moosa HH, Makaroun MS, Peitzman AB, *et al*. TcPO2 values in limb ischemia: effects of blood flow and arterial oxygen tension. J Surg Res. 1986; 40(5): 482–7.

31 Rooke TW, Osmundson PJ. The Influence of age, sex, smoking, and diabetes on lower limb transcutaneous oxygen tension in patients with arterial occlusive disease. Arch Intern Med. 1990; 150: 129–132.

32 Barber FE, Baker DW, Nation AWC, *et al*. Ultrasonic duplex echo-Doppler scanner. IEEE Trans Biomed Eng. 1974; 21: 109.

33 Strandness DE Jr. History of ultrasonic duplex scanning. Cardiovasc Surg. 1996; 4(3): 273–80.

34 Seifert H, Jager K. Diagnostic value of duplex scanning in peripheral vascular disease. Vascular Med Rev. 1990; 1: 21–33.

35 Devine PJ, Carlson DW, Taylor AJ. Clinical value of carotid intima-media thickness testing. J Nucl Cardiol. 2006; 13(5): 710–8.

36 Intersocietal Accreditation Commission. http: //intersocietal.org/vascular/ Accessed: March 2017.

4

Magnetic Resonance, Computed Tomographic, and Angiographic Imaging of Peripheral Artery Disease

Thomas Le[1], Masahiro Horikawa[2] and John A. Kaufman[2]

[1] David Geffen School of Medicine at UCLA, Los Angeles; and Olive View-UCLA Medical Center, Sylmar, CA, USA
[2] Dotter Interventional Institute/Oregon Health & Science University, Portland, OR, USA

Introduction

This chapter describes fundamental aspects of non-invasive and invasive angiography in the evaluation of PAD. Vascular ultrasound is covered in a separate chapter. In the past, physiologic testing and vascular ultrasound represented the standard non-invasive method to screen and evaluate the lower extremities prior to invasive conventional angiography. Cross-sectional imaging with computed tomography angiography (CTA) and magnetic resonance angiography (MRA) has revolutionized this evaluation by helping to determine inflow and outflow arteries and to evaluate the number of lesions, the length of the lesions, lesion diameter and morphology, and the status of the distal runoff. This helps to stratify patients into those who are to receive medical, endovascular, or surgical treatment.

Computed Tomography Angiography

Basics

Computed tomography has its roots in conventional radiography. X-rays are emitted and directed through a body part to be imaged. The X-rays are weakened by the respective densities of the tissues being passed. The remaining X-ray is transmitted to a detector. As opposed to conventional radiography, where there is one emitter and detector, in CT they are an array – an emitter and a detector ring around the patient that can rotate. The collected data are digitized, and used to calculate the X-ray density of the imaged tissue.

Peripheral Artery Disease, Second Edition. Edited by Emile R. Mohler and Michael R. Jaff.
© 2017 John Wiley & Sons Ltd. Published 2017 by John Wiley & Sons Ltd.

Computed tomography angiography became widely available with the advent of multiple rows of detectors (multi-detector CT, MDCT). Single slice detector CT acquires only one slice per rotation, while MDCT can acquire multiple slices per 360° rotation; this improves the speed and resolution of image acquisition. Although much of the original data comparing CTA with digital subtraction angiography (DSA) was based on four-detector row CT, there are eight-, 16-, 64-, 128-, 256-, and even 320-detector row models in widespread clinical use.

Image Acquisition and Interpretation

Protocol
Because the densities of the blood vessels and surrounding soft tissues are similar, iodine-based contrast must be utilized in order to opacify the arteries. The contrast injection protocol is established for each individual scanner, with considerations being injection rate, total volume, and concentration of iodine. Imaging is performed from the diaphragm down to the toes in order to visualize the aorta, visceral arteries, and runoff vessels. Typically, a scout image is first performed. Next, an optional non-contrast acquisition can be performed to evaluate prior stents, blood vessel size, and degree of calcification. A test bolus or bolus triggering series is done subsequently. When the optimal vascular opacification is achieved, the CTA is performed. Often a second optional late phase CTA is done to visualize the venous phase, or sometimes the distal peripheral arteries [1].

Post processing and interpretation. Axial source image review is an important start, as it gives a first impression and also yields critical extravascular anatomy. Simple reformats into coronal and sagittal planes can be helpful for troubleshooting. Thin-slab maximum-intensity projections (MIPs) display the vessels similarly to angiography, although usually without the bones (Figure 4.1b). Volume renderings, on the other hand, preserve three-dimensional (3D) depth information and may show the bones (Figure 4.1c, d). The limitation of both these methods is that vessel calcifications and stents may completely obscure the vascular flow channel [1]. When calcified plaque or stents are present, viewing the data in different planes (i.e., axial, sagittal, coronal), looking at multi-planar reformations, and centerline curved planar reformations at a specialized computer workstation may be helpful.

Figure 4.1 Computed tomography angiography (CTA) of the lower extremities. (a) Axial CTA slice of the proximal thighs shows normal superficial femoral (straight arrow) and profunda femoris (curved arrows) arteries bilaterally. (b) Lower extremity CTA maximum-intensity projection (MIP) demonstrates mild calcific atherosclerotic disease of the distal aorta (arrow), but normal patent vessels distally. (c) Three-dimensional (3D) volume rendering of the same patient without bone. (d) 3D volume rendering with bone. (e) Axial CT in patient with left prosthetic hip (arrow) shows streak artifact, which can make vascular evaluation difficult.

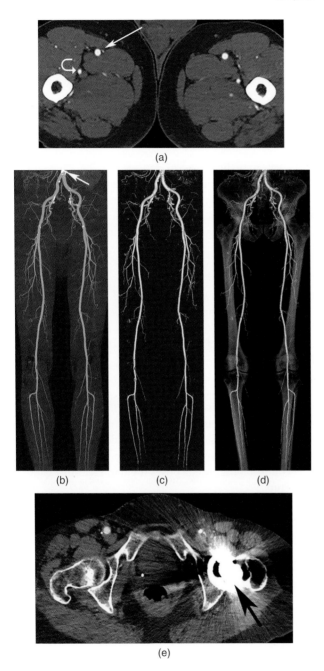

(a)

(b)   (c)   (d)

(e)

Advantages

Multi-detector CT has the fastest image acquisition. A study can be completely acquired in approximately 5 minutes. The whole body can easily be scanned. Furthermore, CT can have a large field of view. MDCT is readily available at imaging centers and hospitals.

Pitfalls

Calcification

Vessel calcification can overestimate the degree of stenosis on CTA. Ouwendijk *et al.* [2] studied 145 patients with CTAs and determined that diabetes, cardiac disease (i.e., history of percutaneous coronary intervention, coronary artery bypass graft, and myocardial infarction), and age > 84 years are independent clinical predictors of vessel calcifications. These patient groups may benefit from alternate forms of imaging.

Artifacts

Along with calcification, dense materials such as metal and bone can obscure vascular structures. This is called beam-hardening or streak artifact; an example of this would be a prosthetic hip or knee (Figure 4.1e). Motion can cause blurring of images, although this is less of a concern compared with magnetic resonance imaging (MRI).

Radiation Exposure

The radiation dose for CTA can quickly escalate due to the multiple scans necessary to perform a study (non-contrast, arterial, delayed, etc.). However, most of the patients with peripheral artery disease (PAD) are older and have a low risk for developing malignancies secondary to the radiation. For pediatric and adolescent patients with a condition that predisposes them to PAD, ultrasound and MRI should be considered.

Contrast-Induced Nephropathy

Contrast-induced nephropathy (CIN) is defined as the impairment of renal function and is calculated as either a 25% increase in serum creatinine from baseline or an absolute increase of 0.5 mg/dL (44 µmol/L) within 48–72 hours of intravenous contrast administration. It is considered by many to be a common cause of iatrogenic acute renal failure; it may be of concern because large doses of contrast are needed to perform CTA exams. Moreover, risk factors for CIN are present in many patients with PAD, such as diabetes, renal insufficiency, congestive heart failure, and anemia [3]. Recently, there has been a debate on the true risk of CIN for patients undergoing CTA, as low-osmolar contrast medium is now in routine use and many of the studies evaluating CIN may not have had optimal study design [4]. If the patient is taking the oral hypoglycemic drug, metformin, the patient should be instructed to wait 48 hours after the CTA before resuming the medication. If the patient has borderline renal insufficiency, the patient's serum creatinine needs to be checked 48 hours after the CTA before metformin is resumed. These are safety measures in order to prevent fatal lactic acidosis [5].

Anaphylaxis

Some patients develop urticaria after contrast injection that is self-limited. True anaphylaxis is rare, occurs shortly after contrast infusion, and is manifested by tachycardia and respiratory distress that quickly become life-threatening. Patients with a history of contrast allergy should receive prophylactic treatment with steroids 24 hours before the scan, with either prednisone or dexamethasone [5]. Diphenhydramine is an optional agent that can help with itchiness and rash.

Magnetic Resonance Angiography

Basics

Magnetic resonance imaging is performed by applying a large external magnetic field to the patient. In addition, applied magnetic field changes (i.e., gradients) and a radiofrequency field (RF, an applied oscillating magnetic field) are employed. These fields magnetize protons in human tissue, which are predominately hydrogen atoms. The contrast of MR images depends on the specific characteristics of the tissue (called T1 and T2) being imaged, and of the specific pulse sequence. The T1 and T2 characteristics can vary depending on the type of tissue, the presence of pathology, or following contrast administration. MR pulse sequences refer to varying combinations of gradients and RF to acquire images. The higher the external field strength, i.e. as one moves from 1.5 to 3 tesla (T), the better the resolution or decreased image time [6].

Image Acquisition and Interpretation

Protocol

The spatial resolution of images is inversely proportional to the image matrix size, and the image matrix size has an impact on the duration of the acquisition; thus, higher-resolution images take longer to acquire. In order to optimize images, different stations of the body are imaged in a stepwise fashion: one for the abdomen/pelvis, thighs, calves, and feet, each with different scanning parameters.

Non-Contrast-Enhanced MRA

Time-of-flight (TOF) angiography has been in widespread clinical use. In this technique, signal is acquired from moving blood by applying RF to a section of tissue, in either a 2D slice or 3D slab fashion. Thus TOF examines blood flow and not the vessel itself. Another non-contrast-enhanced MRA technique that is increasingly employed is electrocardiogram-gated 3D fast spin echo (also known as fresh blood imaging [FBI] and triggered angiography non-contrast-enhanced [TRANCE]), which exploits the flow void effect of fast arterial flow on T2 images. Systolic images, which are dark from fast flow, are subtracted from diastolic images, which are bright from slow flow; the resultant subtracted images are exquisitely sensitive to slow flow and great for peripheral MRA [7–10]. As there is increasing interest in non-contrast imaging, other techniques will probably be adopted in clinical practice in the near future. One example is steady-state free precession (SSFP), which maintains a steady-state longitudinal and transverse magnetization of hydrogen atoms in cells by applying a series of equidistant RF pulses [7]. Techniques such as quiescent-interval single-shot (QISS) MRA and vascular anatomy by non-enhanced static subtraction angiography (VANESSA) are based on SSFP and have had encouraging results [11, 12].

Contrast-Enhanced MRA (CE-MRA)

Magnetic resonance angiography contrast agents are based on gadolinium chelates. Gadolinium contrast makes blood vessels more noticeable on T1 images. Typically, CE-MRA is acquired as a 3D slab. CE-MRA has superior spatial resolution and fewer artifacts compared with TOF imaging, and thus is better to assess stenosis (Figure 4.2) [13]. However, TOF is useful to evaluate the tibial and pedal circulation, particularly if these areas are not well imaged with contrast. In these vessels, TOF may be as accurate as DSA [14].

Post-Processing and Interpretation

As in CTA, source images are first reviewed. Typically, these are the post-contrast images in axial and coronal planes. The source images provide the best resolution and allow artifacts to be easily recognized. MIPs are next reviewed. MRA MIPs display the vessels similar to DSA, though without the bones. Images are made by taking the highest signal intensity in a particular volume. The limitation of MIPs is that when there is complex vascular branching or overlap, it can be difficult to determine the specific path of individual branches, and there can be a tendency to over-grade vessel stenosis [15].

Advantages

Magnetic resonance angiography does not utilize ionizing radiation. Thus, the only penalty for increased image acquisition is time. Gadolinium contrast agents have a lower incidence of anaphylactic reactions than do iodine-based contrast agents. While MR can provide dynamic physiologic imaging in the brain and heart, its applications in PAD are limited. Calcifications can be

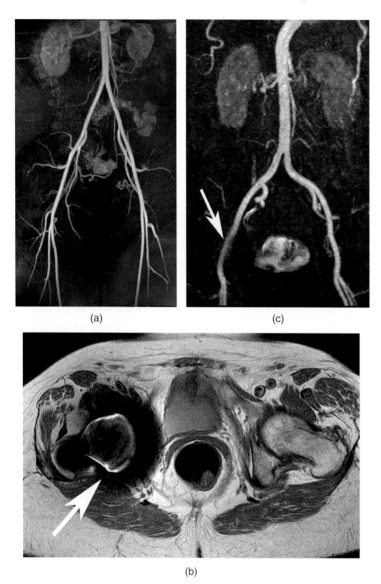

(a)

(c)

(b)

Figure 4.2 Magnetic resonance angiography (MRA) of peripheral arterial disease.
(a) MRA maximum-intensity projection (MIP) image of the distal aorta and pelvis shows normal vascular anatomy and patent vessels without significant stenosis or occlusion.
(b) T1-weighted axial magnetic resonance image demonstrates artifact (arrow) related to right hip prosthesis. (c) MRA of the same patient shows difficulty in evaluating the right common femoral artery related to the artifact from the hip replacement.

considered an advantage or a pitfall, depending on the circumstances. Typically, calcifications cause a signal void. While calcifications do not cause large artifacts in MRA, heavy calcification in smaller vessels may cause artifacts such as apparent stenosis. MRI has exquisite soft tissue contrast, and, in the future, may be useful in evaluating atherosclerotic plaque and determining plaque that is vulnerable to rupture [16, 17].

Pitfalls

Time

Imaging can take approximately 30 minutes. With MRA, there is increased setup time because of patient positioning and data acquisition. The patient needs to be appropriately positioned, as imaging coils need to be placed on the relevant anatomy. During data acquisition, each scan series needs to be set up; furthermore, multiple scans can be performed during the contrast bolus so this can add time.

Nephrogenic Systemic Fibrosis

Nephrogenic systemic fibrosis (NSF) is a debilitating, potentially fatal illness that is observed in patients on dialysis or with severe chronic renal insufficiency (glomerular filtration rate [GFR] < 30mL/min) after receiving gadolinium contrast. Unchelated gadolinium contrast agents, such as gadodiamide (Omniscan) or gadopentetate dimeglumine (Magnevist), are associated with the greatest number of NSF cases. Furthermore, higher-dose contrast studies confer higher risk, such as MRA [5, 18].

Bolus Timing

Although there have been advances in acquisition speed, in many cases there is a small time difference between arterial and venous enhancement. If the acquisition is not timed appropriately for the patient, venous contamination may occur. TOF may be used as a back-up.

Artifacts

Magnetic resonance angiography cannot examine in-stent stenosis as there is metallic artifact. Patients with implanted devices, such as pacemakers and defibrillators, intraocular or intra-aural metallic foreign bodies cannot be imaged (Figure 4.2b, c). It is important to take a thorough history as some newer devices are MRI-safe. If a patient needs monitoring or respiratory equipment for the scan, special non-magnetic equipment is required.

Other Pitfalls

As with CTA, MRA overestimates stenosis. In addition, the bore of the MRI is much smaller than the CT gantry, and many patients become claustrophobic and are unable to complete the scan. While some open MRI systems are available, these typically have low magnetic field strength and are unsuitable for MRA. Behavioral therapy and benzodiazepines have been used with limited success. MRI systems suitable for MRA are not widely available. Another pitfall with MRA is that, because the imaging time is slower, patient motion can make images uninterpretable.

Conventional Angiography

Basics

Lower extremity angiography represents the gold standard examination to evaluate PAD and is now generally reserved for patients in whom an intervention is considered. DSA involves instantaneously subtracting an arterially contrast-enhanced image from a scout image in order to evaluate the vessel lumen. Images can be acquired in subtracted and raw (with bones present) states.

Image Acquisition and Interpretation

Pre-Procedure Patient Care

Inform consent is required, as an invasive procedure is to be performed. Complications of femoral access include hematoma (requiring transfusion, surgery, or delayed discharge; < 0.5%), occlusion (<0.2%), pseudoaneurysm (<0.2%), and arteriovenous fistula (<0.2%) [19]. As the vast majority of patients will need sedation, a physical examination must be performed to categorize patients into the American Society of Anesthesiologists' classification for procedural risk. In addition, a vascular physical examination is necessary to determine patient positioning and access site. Patients' serum laboratory markers need to be checked, including serum creatinine/GFR; the patient may need hydration. Coagulation panel (international normalized ratio [INR] or prothrombin time [PT], activated partial thromboplastin time [aPTT]) and platelet count are other important laboratory tests. An allergy to contrast material should be checked. Anticoagulants such as Coumadin should be discontinued prior to the procedure such that the INR is < 1.5. The patient can be bridged with unfractionated heparin, which is discontinued the night before the procedure. Aspirin and clopidogrel do not need to be held. If the patient has had a serious allergic reaction in the past, the patient should be premedicated with steroids.

Protocol

Patient positioning is dictated typically by the anatomy in question and the access site. Imaging a blood vessel requires multiple frames per second in order to visualize the bolus of contrast as it opacifies the vessel lumen. In addition to recording images in a stationary mode, filming can occur while moving the angiographic table (bolus chase) or rotating the image intensifier/X-ray tube (rotational angiography). Two views of the same vascular structure are typically necessary to evaluate most pathologic processes; en face and orthogonal views are usual. Depending on the vessel location, oblique views from angling the image intensifier/tube may be necessary to display the arterial lumen best (Figure 4.3). Image acquisition and contrast injection protocols have been developed for most vascular anatomies and pathologies. Typically, for PAD, long injections at a lower rate are used in order to completely opacify vessels. Newer rotational angiographic units create datasets that can be used to construct cross-sectional CT-like images and 3D models. Termed cone-beam CT, this technique is a useful troubleshooting tool in evaluating complex vascular anatomy.

Advantages

Digital subtraction angiography can produce exquisite images of the vascular anatomy, with the highest image resolution and image contrast. Unsubtracted images allow the angiographer to see the vascular anatomy superimposed on the bony landmarks. While the cross-sectional modalities can take several "freeze-frames" through an anatomic area of interest, conventional angiography allows for dynamic imaging throughout the arterial phase. Additionally, as arterial access has already been achieved, interventions can be performed and direct pressure measurements obtained.

Pitfalls

Contrast-Induced Nephropathy and Anaphylaxis

As DSA studies use the same contrast material as CTA, patients are at risk for CIN and anaphylactic reactions. Depending on the anatomy in question and the imaging protocol, conventional angiographic study contrast volumes can quickly escalate. It is important to consider the clinical question at the start of the procedure, and limit contrast usage; a general guideline would be to use less than 200 mL per study in an adult patient, but more is often necessary. Unlike in CTA, there are alternative contrast agents available for DSA: carbon dioxide gas (CO_2) and gadolinium chelates. CO_2 has no nephrotoxicity or allergic reaction; it briefly displaces the blood volume in the vessel lumen, resulting in decreased attenuation of the X-ray (negative contrast). A dedicated CO_2 DSA technique must be utilized; typically there is an increased frame rate compared with standard image acquisition (Figure 4.3c). Gadolinium chelates, the intravascular contrast agents for MRA, are another alternative contrast agent; these have a low risk of anaphylaxis. However, patients who have chronic renal insufficiency have a risk for NSF, as stated in the MRA section.

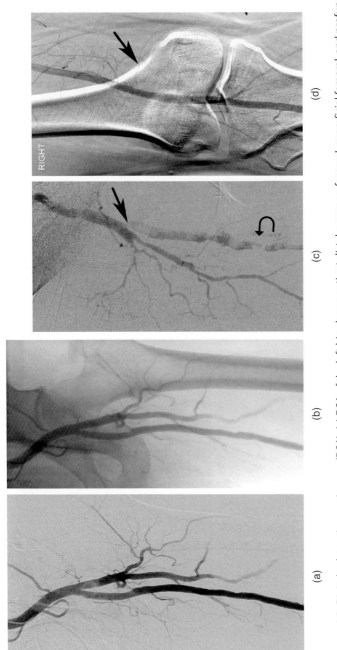

(a)   (b)   (c)   (d)

Figure 4.3 Digital subtraction angiogram (DSA). (a) DSA of the left hip shows patient distal common femoral, superficial femoral, and profunda femoris arteries with mild atherosclerotic disease. The profunda femoris branches are incompletely filled due to the timing of the image. (b) Unsubtracted angiogram of the same study shows the adjacent bone. (c) Carbon dioxide DSA of the right hip shows severe stenosis of the origin of the right superficial femoral artery (arrow), along with multifocal stenosis of the superficial femoral artery (curved arrow). There are also several areas of stenosis in the profunda femoris artery and its branches. (d) DSA of the distal thigh and knee shows motion artifact limiting (arrow) vascular evaluation.

Artifacts

In an uncooperative patient, motion of the extremities can render subtracted images non-diagnostic (Figure 4.3d). Furthermore, in the pelvis, involuntary motion such as bowel peristalsis can make evaluation difficult. Given the ease of obtaining images, radiation dose may accumulate during the course of complex cases. As with contrast use, it is important to contemplate the clinical question at the beginning of the examination and tailor the study appropriately.

Other Disadvantages

Conventional angiography is unable to give information about the vessel wall or plaque. Extravascular structures cannot be visualized.

Intravascular Ultrasonography

Basics

Intravascular ultrasonography (IVUS) is an invasive technology that combines features of non-invasive imaging. IVUS is just like standard ultrasound, in that a probe insonates tissue, and receives reflections from the tissue; this creates the image (Figure 4.4). However, IVUS is unique in that the probe is miniature and is at the end of a catheter. IVUS can assess the vascular lumen, from the inside out. Most IVUS probes are inserted over a guidewire.

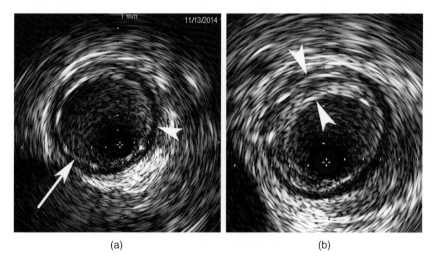

(a)   (b)

Figure 4.4 Intravascular ultrasonography (IVUS) of the lower extremity. (a) Normal IVUS image of the superficial femoral artery showing a normal echogenic intima (arrow) and hypoechoic media (arrowhead). (b) IVUS image shows eccentric intimal plaque (arrowheads) in the superficial femoral artery.

Advantages

Intravascular ultrasonography is a useful adjunct to conventional angiography to take luminal measurements. For instance, in the iliac system, IVUS has been used to determine the appropriate sizing of angioplasty and stent placement; two studies have shown increased patency with IVUS use [20, 21]. Iida *et al.* [22] showed increased patency post-stenting in cases where IVUS was used in the femoropopliteal arteries. IVUS can also be useful to assess intraluminal processes, such as determining plaque distribution and plaque characterization (soft vs. calcified plaque).

Pitfalls

Intravascular ultrasonography probes typically are for single use and this adds cost to the procedure. Most IVUS probes image in the axial plane and so cannot readily provide forward-looking views. A guidewire must already be in place in order to interrogate a vascular territory.

Results

As conventional angiography is considered to be the gold standard, studies are usually compared against this modality. What complicates the data evaluation is that many studies do not list which arterial segments were evaluated. Furthermore, technology is constantly evolving, so it is important to understand what equipment was used in a particular study. The degree of stenosis evaluated and the definitions thereof are additional important variables. While several reviews have pooled data for analysis, these studies have failed to segregate the data. Clinically, this is important in order for one to choose the appropriate type of imaging. Comparison of the visualization of the runoff arteries is difficult, as many studies define the lower extremity runoff differently. For the purposes of this chapter, we have limited our literature review to studies using 16-row MDCT and 1.5 T MRI; on average, these studies were performed in 2008 and afterwards. These data show some improvement compared with a systematic review of the imaging modalities for PAD performed by Collins *et al.* in 2007 [23].

Aortoiliac

CTA

Willmann *et al.* [24], in one of the first studies using 16-row MDCT, prospectively examined 39 patients and defined significant stenosis as greater than 50%. They found 95–99% sensitivity and 98% specificity for aortoiliac disease. Laswed *et al.* [25], in a prospective study of 34 patients using 16-row MDCT, and the same stenosis definition, found 95% sensitivity and 100% specificity. Schernthaner *et al.* [26] published a prospective investigation in 50 patients using 16-row MDCT in which they reported a sensitivity of 100% and specificity of 99.5% for iliac disease. In another prospective study with 50 patients, Albrecht *et al.* [27] found 85–92% sensitivity and 94–100% specificity with 16-row MDCT for aortoiliac. Kau *et al.* [28] more recently used a 64-row MDCT dual-energy system, and in 58 patients found 89% sensitivity and 88% specificity.

MRA

Using a 1.5T CE-MRA in 58 patients, Gjonnaess *et al.* [29] found 96% sensitivity and 94% specificity for aortoiliac occlusive disease, using a definition of significant stenosis of greater than 50%. In a larger retrospective study using 1.5T CE-MRA in 152 patients, Burbelko *et al.* [30] found sensitivity of 73–79% and specificity of 68–81% for significant iliac stenosis defined as greater than 50%. They attributed their results in the pelvic area to overestimation of stenosis grade on MRA [30].

Given that MRA has lower sensitivity and specificity in the pelvis, it may be preferable to utilize CTA in patients without contraindications to radiation or iodinated contrast.

Runoff

CTA

Wilmann *et al.* [24] segregated runoff by femoral disease (sensitivity 97–98%, specificity 94–96%) and popliteal-tibial disease (sensitivity 96–97% and specificity 95–96%). Laswed *et al.* [25] demonstrated sensitivity and specificity of 95% for femoropopliteal disease, and 91% sensitivity and 96% specificity for crural disease. Schernthaner *et al.* [26] showed sensitivity of 97.4% and specificity of 99% for femoral-popliteal disease, and sensitivity of 98.3% and specificity of 99.8% for infra-popliteal disease. Albrecht *et al.*'s [27] results are slightly lower for femoropopliteal disease (sensitivity, 91.5–94.5%; specificity, 94.2–94.9%) and crural disease (sensitivity 89.3–91.8%, specificity 97.7–98.2%). Kau *et al.* [28] found a sensitivity of 67% and specificity of 88% for femoropopliteal disease, and a sensitivity of 91% and specificity of 51% for crural disease.

MRA

Fewer studies examined the runoff vessels compared with CTA. Gjonnaess *et al.* [29] found femoral vessel sensitivity of 92% and specificity of 95%, and popliteal-tibial sensitivity of 93% and specificity of 96%. Deutschmann *et al.* [31] found a sensitivity of 95.6% and specificity of 90.3% for femoropopliteal disease, and a sensitivity of 96.8% and specificity of 96.1% for crural disease. Burbelko *et al.* [30] found a sensitivity of 90-93% and specificity of 89% for femoropopliteal disease, and a sensitivity of 75–89% and specificity of 64–68% for crural disease.

Throughout the runoff vessels, CTA and MRA have similar results, with average sensitivities and specificities > 90%. Kau *et al.* [28] noted decreased diagnostic accuracy in the calf vessels for CTA, although their study primarily evaluated MIP images only. Only one reader was allowed to use axial images, and only for troubleshooting difficult segments. The Kau protocol does not follow what is routinely done in clinical practice, where axial images are the mainstay of diagnosis. For MRA, the Burbelko group noted that the MRA diagnostic accuracy was decreased due to uninterpretable studies. In the end, it is likely the CTA and MRA are similarly acceptable for the runoff vessels, if the study is of high quality. CTA and MRA both suffer when there are heavily calcified vessels in the calf, as well as when there is venous contamination.

Pedal

CTA

Laswed *et al.* [25] reported a sensitivity of 100% and specificity of 90% for the pedal vessels. Albrecht *et al.* [27] achieved a sensitivity of 92% and specificity of 97%. Kau *et al.* [28] had less impressive results, with a sensitivity of 85% and specificity of 18%.

MRA

Only one study during the period under consideration examined the pedal vessels using MRA. Kos *et al.* [32] examined 20 patients in a CE-MRA 1.5T based system, and found a sensitivity of 91.4% and a specificity of 96.1%.

There are limited studies evaluating the pedal vessels specifically, but more CTA studies have been performed. At this time, either modality is probably acceptable.

Conclusion

High-resolution and high-contrast images can be obtained with non-invasive CTA and MRA in evaluating patients for PAD. This helps to stratify patients into those who are to receive medical, endovascular, or surgical treatment. For patients undergoing endovascular procedures, satisfactory cross-sectional imaging allows a more directed intervention.

References

1 Fleischmann D, Hallett RL, Rubin GD. CT angiography of peripheral arterial disease. J Vasc Intervent Radiol. 2006; 17(1): 3–26.

2 Ouwendijk R, Kock MC, van Dijk LC, *et al.* Vessel wall calcifications at multi-detector row CT angiography in patients with peripheral arterial disease: effect on clinical utility and clinical predictors. Radiology. 2006; 241(2): 603–8.

3 Golshahi J, Nasri H, Gharipour M. Contrast-induced nephropathy; A literature review. J Nephropathol. 2014; 3(2): 51–6.

4 Davenport MS, Cohan RH, Khalatbari S, Ellis JH. The challenges in assessing contrast-induced nephropathy: where are we now? Am J Roentgenol. 2014; 202(4): 784–9.

5 American College of Radiology. ACR Manual on Contrast Media, v10.2, 2016. Online: https://www.acr.org/~/media/ACR/Documents/PDF/QualitySafety/Resources/Contrast-Manual/2016_Contrast_Media.pdf?la=en. Accessed: March 2017.

6 McRobbie DW. MRI from Picture to Proton, 2 edn. Cambridge: Cambridge University Press, 2007.

7 Morita S, Masukawa A, Suzuki K, *et al.* Unenhanced MR Angiography: Techniques and Clinical Applications in Patients with Chronic Kidney Disease. Radiographics. 2011; 31(2): E13–33.

8 Lim RP, Hecht EM, Xu J, *et al.* 3D nongadolinium-enhanced ECG-gated MRA of the distal lower extremities: preliminary clinical experience. J Magn Reson Im. 2008; 28(1): 181–9.

9 Gutzeit A, Sutter R, Froehlich JM, *et al.* ECG-triggered non-contrast-enhanced MR angiography (TRANCE) versus digital subtraction angiography (DSA) in patients with peripheral arterial occlusive disease of the lower extremities. Eur Radiol. 2011; 21(9): 1979–87.

10 Mohrs OK, Petersen SE, Heidt MC, *et al.* High-resolution 3D non-contrast-enhanced, ECG-gated, multi-step MR angiography of the lower extremities: comparison with contrast-enhanced MR angiography. Eur Radiol. 2011; 21(2): 434–42.

11 Hodnett PA, Koktzoglou I, Davarpanah AH, *et al.* Evaluation of peripheral arterial disease with nonenhanced quiescent-interval single-shot MR angiography. Radiology. 2011; 260(1): 282–93.

12 Priest AN, Joubert I, Winterbottom AP, *et al.* Initial clinical evaluation of a non-contrast-enhanced MR angiography method in the distal lower extremities. Magn Reson Med. 2013; 70(6): 1644–52.

13 Met R, Bipat S, Legemate DA, *et al.* Diagnostic performance of computed tomography angiography in peripheral arterial disease: a systematic review and meta-analysis. JAMA. 2009; 301(4): 415–24.

14 McCauley TR, Monib A, Dickey KW, *et al.* Peripheral vascular occlusive disease: accuracy and reliability of time-of-flight MR angiography. Radiology. 1994; 192(2): 351–7.

15 Rubin GD, Rofsky NM. CT and MR Angiography: Comprehensive Vascular Assessment. Lippincott Williams & Wilkins, 2008.

16 Isbell DC, Meyer CH, Rogers WJ, *et al*. Reproducibility and reliability of atherosclerotic plaque volume measurements in peripheral arterial disease with cardiovascular magnetic resonance. J Cardiovasc Magn Reson. 2007; 9(1): 71–6.

17 Li F, McDermott MM, Li D, *et al*. The association of lesion eccentricity with plaque morphology and components in the superficial femoral artery: a high-spatial-resolution, multi-contrast weighted CMR study. J Cardiovasc Magn Reson. 2010; 12: 37.

18 Broome DR, Girguis MS, Baron PW, *et al*. Gadodiamide-associated nephrogenic systemic fibrosis: why radiologists should be concerned. Am J Roentgenol. 2007; 188(2): 586–92.

19 Singh H, Cardella JF, Cole PE, *et al*. Quality improvement guidelines for diagnostic arteriography. J Vasc Intervent Radiol. 2003; 14(9 Pt 2): S283–8.

20 Buckley CJ, Arko FR, Lee S, *et al*. Intravascular ultrasound scanning improves long-term patency of iliac lesions treated with balloon angioplasty and primary stenting. J Vasc Surg. 2002; 35(2): 316–23.

21 Ichihashi S, Higashiura W, Itoh H, *et al*. Intravascular ultrasound assessment of acute expansion of the balloon-expandable stent in heavy calcified iliac artery lesions or in lesions resistant to dilation by a self-expanding stent. Ann Vasc Surg. 2014; 28(6): 1449–55.

22 Iida O, Takahara M, Soga Y, *et al*. Efficacy of intravascular ultrasound in femoropopliteal stenting for peripheral artery disease with TASC II Class A to C Lesions. J Endovasc Ther. 2014; 21(4): 485–92.

23 Collins R, Burch J, Cranny G, *et al*. Duplex ultrasonography, magnetic resonance angiography, and computed tomography angiography for diagnosis and assessment of symptomatic, lower limb peripheral arterial disease: systematic review. BMJ. 2007; 334(7606): 1257.

24 Willmann JK, Baumert B, Schertler T, *et al*. Aortoiliac and lower extremity arteries assessed with 16-detector row CT angiography: prospective comparison with digital subtraction angiography. Radiology. 2005; 236(3): 1083–93.

25 Laswed T, Rizzo E, Guntern D, *et al*. Assessment of occlusive arterial disease of abdominal aorta and lower extremities arteries: value of multidetector CT angiography using an adaptive acquisition method. Eur Radiol. 2008; 18(2): 263–72.

26 Schernthaner R, Stadler A, Lomoschitz F, *et al*. Multidetector CT angiography in the assessment of peripheral arterial occlusive disease: accuracy in detecting the severity, number, and length of stenoses. Eur Radiol. 2008; 18(4): 665–71.

27 Albrecht T, Foert E, Holtkamp R, *et al*. 16-MDCT angiography of aortoiliac and lower extremity arteries: comparison with digital subtraction angiography. Am J Roentgenol. 2007; 189(3): 702–11.

28 Kau T, Eicher W, Reiterer C, *et al.* Dual-energy CT angiography in peripheral arterial occlusive disease-accuracy of maximum intensity projections in clinical routine and subgroup analysis. Eur Radiol. 2011; 21(8): 1677–86.

29 Gjonnaess E, Morken B, Sandbaek G, *et al.* Gadolinium-enhanced magnetic resonance angiography, colour duplex and digital subtraction angiography of the lower limb arteries from the aorta to the tibio-peroneal trunk in patients with intermittent claudication. Eur J Vasc Endovasc Surg. 2006; 31(1): 53–8.

30 Burbelko M, Augsten M, Kalinowski MO, Heverhagen JT. Comparison of contrast-enhanced multi-station MR angiography and digital subtraction angiography of the lower extremity arterial disease. J Magn Reson Im. 2013; 37(6): 1427–35.

31 Deutschmann HA, Schoellnast H, Portugaller HR, *et al.* Routine use of three-dimensional contrast-enhanced moving-table MR angiography in patients with peripheral arterial occlusive disease: comparison with selective digital subtraction angiography. Cardiovasc Inter Rad. 2006; 29(5): 762–70.

32 Kos S, Reisinger C, Aschwanden M, *et al.* Pedal angiography in peripheral arterial occlusive disease: first-pass i.v. contrast-enhanced MR angiography with blood pool contrast medium versus intraarterial digital subtraction angiography. Am J Roentgenol. 2009; 192(3): 775–84.

5

Non-atherosclerotic Peripheral Artery Disease

Mitchell D. Weinberg[1] and Ido Weinberg[2]

[1] Northwell Health System; and Hofstra Northwell School of Medicine, Long Island, NY, USA
[2] Massachusetts General Hospital, Boston, MA, USA

Introduction – Presentation of Peripheral Artery Disease

The presentation and clinical manifestations of atherosclerosis in the lower extremities are termed peripheral artery disease (PAD). Thus, risk of developing PAD mirrors classic atherosclerotic risk factors such as tobacco abuse, hypertension, and hyperlipidemia. It is a common condition, affecting 4.3–29% of the adult population – this percentage increases with patient age and as other vascular beds are affected [1, 2]. Clinically, PAD is usually asymptomatic; however, it may present with lower extremity symptoms. While the "classical" presentation is often recognized as cramping calf pain that is exacerbated by activity, and promptly relieved by rest, most symptomatic patients actually present with "atypical" leg symptoms. These may manifest as differing qualities of pain (e.g., tingling, burning etc.) and different locations of pain (e.g., thighs, buttocks). Also, some patients with PAD present with critical limb ischemia (CLI) – this is the term used to describe patients who suffer rest pain, ulcerations or gangrene.

While most patients who present with lower extremity pain with exertion are eventually diagnosed with PAD, in some the diagnosis is not related to atherosclerosis. This group of uncommon entities is collectively known as non-atherosclerotic peripheral artery disease (NAPAD). Unfortunately, due to their rarity, these conditions are frequently overlooked, misdiagnosed or mismanaged, leading to unfortunate and preventable adverse outcomes [3]. These conditions share some clinical characteristics with PAD, while differing in others, and should be considered as part of the differential diagnosis of any patient with leg pain with exertion. The following sections will outline when to suspect

Peripheral Artery Disease, Second Edition. Edited by Emile R. Mohler and Michael R. Jaff.
© 2017 John Wiley & Sons Ltd. Published 2017 by John Wiley & Sons Ltd.

NAPAD and will offer a rational clinical approach to patients with leg pain with exertion.

Premature lower extremity atherosclerosis (PLEA) is a subtype of PAD that merits specific attention in this regard. At first glance, PLEA may raise the suspicion of a non-atherosclerotic underlying condition as the source of a patient's complaints. However, as in PAD, the etiology of pathology in PLEA is atherosclerosis and therefore evaluation and treatment should be the same [4].

When Should Non-atherosclerotic Causes of PAD Be Suspected?

Cardiovascular and primary care physicians routinely encounter patients who present with leg pain with exertion. Clearly, most of these patients are diagnosed with PAD. However, other clinical entities must not be overlooked, as misdiagnosing NAPAD may result in patient mismanagement and poor clinical outcomes (Figure 5.1). The differentiation of NAPAD from PAD should rely on a gestalt of symptoms, imaging patterns and key laboratory findings. Proper diagnosis is often a matter of clinical suspicion and pattern recognition (Table 5.1).

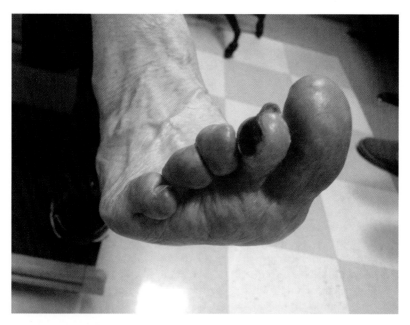

Figure 5.1 Necrotic ulcer on the lateral aspect of the second toe of the right foot ("kissing toe ulcer") in a patient with peripheral artery disease and critical limb ischemia.

Table 5.1 Comparison of atherosclerosis and non-atherosclerotic peripheral artery disease (NAPAD).

Characteristics	Age at presentation	Anatomic distribution	Inflammatory markers	Systemic organ involvement	Imaging characteristics	Unique features/manifestations
Atherosclerosis	Older, usually > 50 years	Typical location: – artery ostium – multi-vessel involvement – lesions of variable lengths	Variable. Not typically elevated –elevated inflammatory markers (hs-CRP); associated with increased risk of systemic cardiovascular events and mortality	Multiple vascular beds are often involved	Lesion characteristics vary by anatomical location: – focal at internal iliac artery origin – diffuse in superficial femoral artery – occlusion common in superficial femoral artery	Increased prevalence of coronary and cerebrovascular disease in patients with lower extremity PAD
NAPAD	Usually younger than atherosclerosis; however, varies according to etiology	Variable location; examples are: – popliteal: cystic adventitial disease – renal and carotid: FMD – mid-aortic/ great vessels: in Takayasu's arteritis	Depending on the etiology; however, elevated in vasculitis and atheromatous embolization	Variable such as: – arteritis: skin, kidneys, brain – FMD: renal and carotids	Unique findings such as: – "halo" sign in Takayasu's; – arterial "beading" in most common form of FMD (medial fibroplasias) – intraluminal defect in cystic adventitial disease – dynamic findings – arterial stenosis with provocative maneuvers (PAES)	Arterial 'beading – FMD Peri-arterial inflammation – arteritis Elevated compartment pressures – exertional compartment syndrome Development of arterial stenosis with limb positions – endofibrosis, popliteal artery entrapment syndrome Abnormal Allen's test – Buerger's disease

PAD, peripheral artery disease; FMD, fibromuscular dysplasia; hs-CRP, high-sensitivity C-reactive protein; PAES, popliteal artery entrapment syndrome.

First, there is the typical presentation. Patients with PAD are often older, as PAD is correlated with other cardiovascular disease. Presentation at a younger age, while potentially a result of PLEA or Post-irradiation accelerated atherosclerosis, may be a telltale sign of NAPAD.

Next, classically symptomatic patients with PAD complain of cramping calf pain that is exacerbated by activity and is worse when walking on uneven surfaces and on an incline. The pain will usually start at a given time for a particular patient and does not usually occur at rest or with standing (i.e., without walking). Symptoms will usually be relieved within 5–10 minutes after the patient rests and sitting is usually not necessary to relieve the pain. Atypical symptoms should prompt the astute clinician to consider another diagnosis as the cause of the patient's complaints. Atypical symptoms may differ from the above-mentioned classical presentation in one or several elements. Examples include differing triggers (e.g., leg pain that only occurs after maximal exertion in a young athlete), lagging pain resolution, atypical pain characteristics or location and pain that may also appear while the patient is standing still.

The next clue to the diagnosis of NAPAD are imaging findings (Figure 5.2). Atherosclerotic PAD is characterized by involvement of multiple vascular beds. In other words, isolated PAD is atypical. Also, lesions are often of variable length and are associated with calcifications (Figure 5.3). Atypical imaging findings may include arterial wall thickening, variation with maneuvers, periarterial cysts and arterial malformations typical of fibromuscular dysplasia.

Finally, atherosclerosis is associated with cardiovascular risk factors. Thus, patients presenting with PAD will often have abused tobacco, have an abnormal lipid profile and may suffer from diabetes mellitus. However, it is uncommon for PAD patients to present with elevated inflammatory markers. On the other hand, some subtypes of NAPAD (e.g., vasculitis) may present with elevation of markers of inflammation such as erythrocyte sedimentation rate or C-reactive protein.

In patients in whom any of the above-mentioned characteristics of PAD are not present, a diagnosis of NAPAD should at least be entertained.

Entities that Make up Non-atherosclerotic PAD

The following sections describe the presentation, diagnosis (Table 5.1) and treatment (Table 5.2) of various conditions that make up NAPAD.

Popliteal Artery Entrapment Syndrome

Popliteal artery entrapment syndrome (PAES) usually presents as intermittent claudication in younger individuals and is more often described in men than in women [5]. It results from pressure exerted on the popliteal artery, and sometimes the popliteal vein, by muscles or ligaments in the popliteal fossa [6]. The

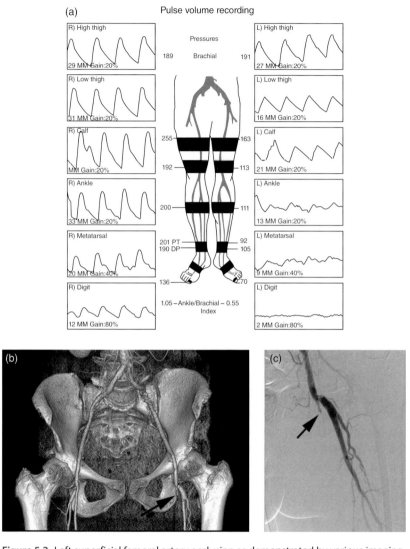

Figure 5.2 Left superficial femoral artery occlusion as demonstrated by various imaging modalities. (a) Segmental pressure measurements demonstrating reduced pressures in both the upper and lower thigh cuffs compared with the right lower extremity and brachial pressure cuffs. Pulse volume recordings revealing moderate disease at the thigh level. (b) Computed tomography three-dimensional reconstruction demonstrating total occlusion of the superficial femoral artery on the left near its origin (arrow). (c) Digital subtraction angiography demonstrating total occlusion of the superficial femoral artery on the left near its origin (arrow).

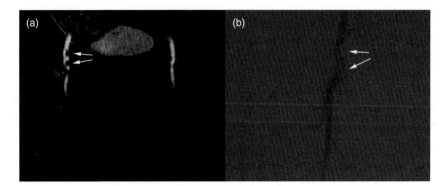

Figure 5.3 Appearance of common femoral artery plaque in two imaging modalities. (a) Magnetic resonance angiography demonstrating two discrete, calcific stenoses in the common femoral artery (arrows). (b) Digital subtraction angiography demonstrating common femoral artery stenoses corresponding to the findings in (a) (arrows).

Table 5.2 Treatment of non-atherosclerotic peripheral artery disease (NAPAD).

Entity	Elements of treatment	Comments
Peripheral artery disease	Cardiovascular risk factor optimization, lifestyle modification, exercise (preferably supervised). Consider endovascular and surgical intervention	Intervention should typically be offered to patients suffering from lifestyle-limiting intermittent claudication or critical limb ischemia
Popliteal artery entrapment syndrome	Surgical release of the entrapment. Sometimes bypass of a degenerative aneurysm is needed	
External iliac artery endofibrosis	Most commonly surgical. Stenting has been described	
Fibromuscular dysplasia	Medical therapy should probably consist of an antiplatelet agent and blood pressure control. Intervention with angioplasty (without stenting) may be preferable to stenting when necessary	Limited high-quality data. Most treatments are empirical
Exertional compartment syndrome	Physical therapy, exercise modification. Fasciotomy in select cases	
Cystic adventitial disease	Excision of cysts	Cyst drainage is usually not durable
Vasculitis	For active disease – immune modulating treatment	Strictures ("burnt out" disease) may require surgery or endovascular intervention
Musculoskeletal pathology	Condition-specific	

prevalence of PAES is probably very low, and was described in as few as 33 of approximately 20 000 Greek military recruits (0.17%) [7]. The diagnosis may be complicated by the fact that findings of anatomic "entrapment" (as opposed to symptoms) are actually not uncommon [8]. PAES is divided into four types (I–IV) in which there is arterial compression; type V, in which the popliteal vein is also involved; and type VI, which is functional, a result of a hypertrophied medial head of the gastrocnemius muscle [9].

Symptoms of PAES include pain, paresthesias and cold feet after exercise. Left neglected ischemic rest pain and tissue necrosis may develop. These symptoms are less common and result from arterial degeneration and post-stenotic aneurysmal dilatation which may result in acute arterial occlusion or distal athero-embolization. Paradoxically, in long-standing cases, well-developed arterial collaterals may actually result in milder symptoms. Notably, bilateral symptoms have been described [5]. If the popliteal vein is involved, leg swelling, heaviness, varicosities and nocturnal calf cramps may develop [10].

The diagnosis of PAES is suggested by examining the popliteal pulse twice – once while the patient is in the neutral position and once with maneuvers. Popliteal blood flow should also be tested by a continuous Doppler signal when the probe is placed over the distal tibial arteries. The popliteal pulse will diminish or disappear with active plantarflexion against resistance. This is a result of popliteal artery compression. Surprisingly, this is not always an easy diagnostic maneuver to perform. Another useful study comprises pulse volume recordings and segmental pressures measured at rest with the knee extended and the ankle in the neutral, dorsiflexed and plantarflexed positions. Adding exercise may be helpful as well. Next, arterial duplex ultrasonography (DUS) may demonstrate abnormalities when performed in the aforementioned positions [11]. However, it should be noted that in a series of 16 healthy volunteers, popliteal artery compression was demonstrated in 84% of limbs upon active plantarflexion, highlighting the potential for false-positive results [12]. As physiological, bedside testing is frustrating and difficult to interpret, dynamic computerized tomographic arteriography (CTA) or magnetic resonance arteriography (MRA) or even contrast angiography are often used to confirm the diagnosis. A benefit of CTA and MRA is that they can actually demonstrate the structures resulting in entrapment of the vascular structures. Unfortunately, data regarding the utility of these tests are limited to small series [13].

Treatment of PAES is surgical relief of the entrapment by resection or translocation of the compressing elements. This is also true in the case of functional PAES, in which part of the medial head of the gastrocnemius muscle is resected to relieve pressure [9]. Therapy should not be delayed, to avoid long-term consequences of the disorder (Figure 5.4). Nonetheless, if the disease is advanced, arterial reconstruction or surgical bypass of an occlusion or aneurysm may be needed.

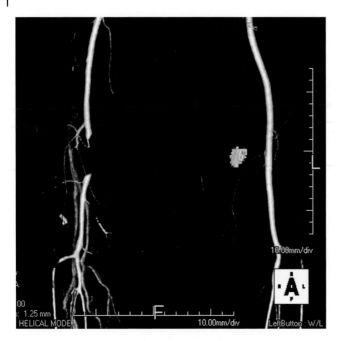

Figure 5.4 Computed tomography demonstrating total occlusion of the right popliteal artery in a patient with longstanding untreated popliteal artery entrapment syndrome.

External Iliac Artery Endofibrosis

External iliac artery endofibrosis (EIAE) is a unique cause of intermittent claudication described exclusively in highly competitive athletes (e.g., cyclists, runners, triathletes and speed skaters). There is very little published on EIAE, but some have estimated its prevalence to be as high as 20% in elite cyclists [14]. The pathophysiology of this condition is not well delineated; however, the end result is narrowing of the external iliac artery lumen by subendothelial deposition of fibrous tissue. Patients typically describe cramps in their calves or thighs that appear at near maximal effort and mandate cessation of activity. Other symptoms may include a sensation of fullness or numbness. Symptoms usually resolve upon cessation of activity; however, progression to bilateral external iliac artery occlusion has been described.

If EIAE is suspected, physical examination should focus on eliciting femoral bruits with hip flexion [15]. Cycling ergometry and tailored exercise testing should follow. Imaging studies, including CTA and MRA, may show subtle narrowing of the external iliac artery.

Treatment of EIAE has classically been surgical. Surgical options include endofibrectomy, patch angioplasty and bypass grafting and may also combine shortening of redundant artery [15]. Endovascular therapy has also been described. Angioplasty is considered insufficient, and stent placement is central for achieving long-term patency [16].

Fibromuscular Dysplasia

Fibromuscular dysplasia (FMD) is an oft-neglected non-atherosclerotic, noninflammatory arteriopathy of unknown etiology and debatable prevalence that may involve any arterial bed [17, 18]. It is more common in women than in men, and the mean age of diagnosis is 52 years [19]. Most patients with FMD are probably asymptomatic, and hypertension is the most common clinical manifestation in symptomatic patients. However FMD can mimic PAD when it involves the aorta or arteries of the lower extremities [11]. One way to characterize FMD is according to which arterial layer is affected, and another is according to the arteriographic pattern of disease [20]. Medial fibroplasia is the most common type, comprising 80–90% of cases and obstruction to flow results from intra-arterial webs.

The diagnosis of FMD is often based on typical imaging findings. The characteristic "string of beads" appearance of medial fibroplasia can sometimes be seen with duplex, but the diagnosis is often confirmed with more advanced imaging techniques [21] (Figure 5.5). A definitive diagnosis can be fortified with pathology, but tissue is rarely available. Angiography and intravascular ultrasound are considered the gold standard diagnostic modalities [22] but are also often not performed given their invasive nature. The differential diagnosis

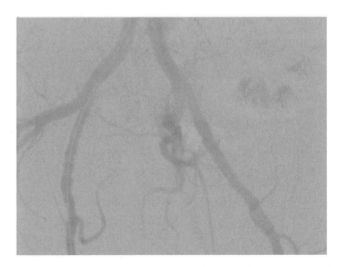

Figure 5.5 Digital subtraction angiography of the iliac arteries showing the characteristic "string of beads" appearance of medial fibroplasias fibromuscular dysplasia bilaterally, more evident on the right.

of FMD includes not only atherosclerosis, but also systemic vasculitis, segmental arterial mediolysis (SAM) [23] and arterial aneurysms and dissections from other causes such as Ehlers–Danlos IV or Marfan syndrome [24]. Given the median age of diagnosis, coexisting atherosclerosis is not uncommon.

Treatment of FMD should be tailored to patient symptoms and the affected vascular bed. Patients who have renal or carotid artery involvement should undergo imaging of their brain vasculature, as a relatively high prevalence of intracranial aneurysms has been described. Medical therapy for this condition has empirically included aspirin; however, there are few objective data to support this practice. Medical therapy should also target end-organ effects of reduced blood flow. A common example includes treatment of hypertension in patients with renal artery FMD. In the context of NAPAD, intervention is rarely needed in patients who suffer limiting symptoms. In such cases, angioplasty without stenting is preferred, as inferred from data originating from renal artery interventions [25].

Cystic Adventitial Disease

Cystic adventitial disease (CAD) is related to arterial compression by external cysts (Figure 5.6). It typically affects middle-aged men. The origin of the cysts is unclear. Various theories have been proposed for the etiology of CAD, including a systemic disorder, repetitive trauma, and a persistent embryonic synovial track [26]. This condition has been described most commonly as affecting the popliteal artery; however, other vascular beds have been identified, as well as bilateral disease [27].

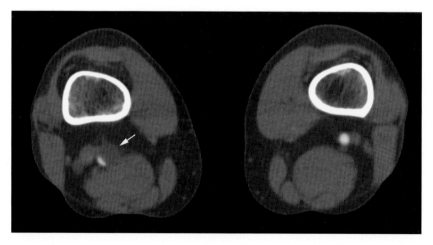

Figure 5.6 Computed tomography demonstrating a cyst compressing the right popliteal artery (arrow) in a patient with cystic adventitial disease.

Symptoms are classically intermittent and may wax and wane over time. Typically, resting will result in resolution of pain after longer periods of time than in PAD, often over a period of 20 minutes [28]. Physical examination in CAD should include an attempt to elicit the Ishikawa sign; disappearance of pedal pulses with knee flexion. Imaging should aim at identifying the cysts. This may be achieved with duplex, but magnetic resonance imaging is often more reliable. It is noteworthy that digital subtraction angiography is actually not the gold standard diagnostic modality for CAD, as it may only demonstrate compression of the arterial lumen ("hourglass sign") without further characterization of the etiology [29].

Treatment of CAD consists of excision of the offending cysts, as aspiration alone may result in recurrence. Occluded segments should be bypassed [30].

Vasculitis

Vasculitis is often divided to small-, medium-, and large-artery vasculitis. The vasculitis that mimics PAD is most likely large-vessel vasculitis and especially Takayasu's arteritis (TA).

Takayasu's arteritis affects mainly young women of Asian descent. Other variants have been described in Indian men [31] and in women of Latin descent. In the context of intermittent claudication, a mid-aortic variant of TA may manifest with diminished flow to the lower extremities as a result of aortic coarctation [32]. This presentation is uncommon, affecting only 41 in a series of 272 TA patients [33]. Symptoms may arise during active phases of the disease, but also from impingement of flow secondary to scarring, in the so called "burnt out" phases of the disease [34]. Thus, when implicating TA as the cause of a patient's symptoms, inflammatory markers are not necessarily elevated.

Criteria for the diagnosis of TA include young age, claudication of more than one extremity, a decreased brachial pulse, an inter-brachial systolic blood pressure difference > 10 mmHg, a bruit over at least one subclavian artery and imaging evidence of narrowing of the aorta or one of its large branches [35]. As noted, elevated inflammatory markers are not necessary for the diagnosis. Typical duplex findings in TA include arterial wall edema ("halo sign" [36]) and arterial narrowing ("spaghetti sign" [37]) (Figure 5.7). Long-segment narrowing as well as aneurysmal changes may be diagnosed with CTA or MRA [38]. Positron emission CT (PET-CT) should be used with caution, as uptake may lag treatment initiation considerably [39, 40].

Treatment of TA should address inflammation, arterial complications and systemic complications (e.g., myositis) [41]. Inflammation is usually controlled with the use of corticosteroids, methotrexate and the anti-interleukin-6 agent, tocilizumab [42]. Arterial narrowing that results in symptoms can be addressed with endovascular techniques, while aneurysms may require open surgical intervention. Rarely bypass grafting is necessary.

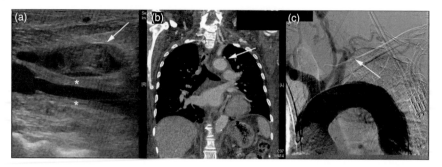

Figure 5.7 Takayasu's arteritis. (a) Duplex image of a common carotid artery demonstrating long segment wall thickening (asterisks) and an incidental finding of internal jugular vein thrombosis (arrow). (b) A thickened aortic wall (arrow) as seen on computed tomographic angiography. (c) Left subclavian artery occlusion and collateral flow (arrow) as seen on digital subtraction angiography.

Idiopathic Mid-aortic Syndrome

Mid-aortic syndrome is a form of aortic coarctation that is different than involvement of the aorta in a systemic vasculitis. It most probably arises from an embryonic developmental disorder or from a genetically mediated process, and is typically diagnosed in children and young adults [43]. Mid-aortic syndrome can affect the distal thoracic (distal to the ligamentum arteriosum), suprarenal, renal, or infrarenal segments of the abdominal aorta, and intermittent claudication has been described, albeit rarely [44]. Treatment of mid-aortic syndrome has classically been surgery [45], because of a high reported recurrence rate with percutaneous transluminal angioplasty, possibly owing to extensive aortic involvement and significant elastic recoil. Stenting may have a potential role in treatment of these unusual patients.

Arterial Manifestations of Pseudoxanthoma Elasticum

Pseudoxanthoma elasticum (PXE) is a rare autosomal recessive inherited multisystem disease that results in ectopic mineralization of elastic tissue [46]. The causative mutation is usually in the gene encoding for the ATP-binding cassette transporter C6 (ABCC6) [47] and the full extent of the phenotype is usually not apparent until the second or third decade of life. While intermittent claudication [48] and CLI [49] are not central to the clinical presentation of PXE patients, mineralization of mid-sized arteries in the extremities can occur. The astute clinician will need to notice other clinical manifestations in order to suspect PXE. In the skin, small yellowish papules usually appear in flexion areas, including the neck, and antecubital and popliteal fossae. In the eyes, patients with PXE have angioid streaks and later ocular hemorrhages. Gastrointestinal bleeding, especially from a diffusely friable gastric mucosa, is a dreaded manifestation of PXE and can be life-threatening and precede other manifestations of the disease [50, 51].

Reports concerning the treatment of peripheral manifestations of PXE are scarce but include surgery [52] and percutaneous transluminal angioplasty [53]. Importantly, aspirin should be avoided because of the life-threatening risk of gastrointestinal hemorrhage.

Chronic Exertional Compartment Syndrome

The calf is divided into four anatomical compartments. Chronic exertional compartment syndrome (CECS) refers to activity-related, reversible, pressure elevation in one or more of these compartments. The rise in pressure results in reduced tissue perfusion and neuromuscular dysfunction [54]. While not vascular, the symptom pattern of this condition makes it important for the cardiovascular specialist to recognize, as it is part of the differential diagnosis of exertional leg pain.

Chronic exertional compartment syndrome usually affects young athletes such as runners or basketball players [55]. Early symptoms include pain or burning over the affected compartment, and in more advanced cases presentation involves paresthesias and weakness. The location of discomfort is not an accurate localizer of the specific limb compartments involved, and direct measurements are necessary for an accurate diagnosis [56].

Patients who are diagnosed with CECS often have multiple imaging studies performed before the diagnosis is suspected and confirmed [57]. This stems from the fact that the diagnosis of CECS must include intra-compartmental pressure measurements before and during exercise. These are best performed by specially trained orthopedic surgeons and can be done in the office setting by a handheld manometer [58].

A two-step approach is usually utilized in the treatment of CECS. First, training regimen alterations, footwear optimization and physical therapy are tried. If these fail, controlled fasciotomy may be necessary to allow return to activity. Recovery is usually expected within several weeks.

Musculoskeletal Pathology

Much common musculoskeletal pathology may produce leg pain upon exertion that can mimic PAD and CLI. Examples of such conditions include tight hamstring muscles, plantar fasciitis and acute and chronic arthritis of various causes. As these conditions are variable in presentation, so are patient and symptom characteristics. Further complicating the diagnosis is the fact that many patients have concomitant atherosclerotic risk factors, as some types of musculoskeletal disease are more common with advanced age. Therefore, these diagnoses are usually made on the basis of excellent physical examination as a result of a high level of clinical suspicion. Ruling out a significant vascular contribution may also be useful.

Diagnostic Evaluation of Patients with Leg Pain with Exertion

The diagnosis of each NAPAD has been described in detail in previous sections. This section offers an overview of the approach to diagnosis of exertional leg pain as a whole. As with most other complex medical diagnoses, the approach in patients presenting with leg pain with exertion should follow the familiar pattern of thorough history and comprehensive physical examination fortified by appropriate maneuvers. Focused laboratory and imaging studies should follow and should result from specific pre-test probability. Figure 5.8 suggests a diagnostic approach in patients presenting with leg pain with exertion.

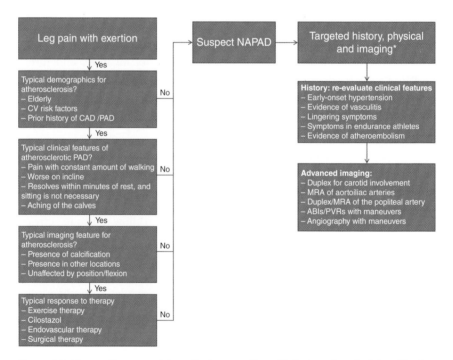

Figure 5.8 Diagnostic approach to patients presenting with lower extremity intermittent claudication. *Refer to Table 5.1 for more details. NAPAD, non-atherosclerotic peripheral artery disease; CAD, cystic adventitial disease; PAD, peripheral artery disease; MRA, magnetic resonance arteriography; ABI, ankle–brachial index; PVR, pulse volume recording.

Treatment Considerations

The treatment of individual NAPAD conditions is described in previous sections and summarized in Table 5.2. This section summarizes the treatment approach to NAPAD as a whole. In general terms, a treatment plan of any patient with PAD should include lifestyle interventions, medical therapy, exercise and, in certain patients, intervention [59]. Intervention may be endovascular or surgical. Similarly, NAPAD patients should also be offered a combination of conservative measures and judiciously selected intervention. However, entity-specific modifications should also be part of any NAPAD treatment plan, thus highlighting the importance of appropriate diagnosis and management (Figure 5.2).

Perhaps surprisingly, despite the high prevalence of patients presenting with leg pain with exertion, there is a knowledge gap regarding the optimal medical therapy they should be offered. Nonetheless, standard of care typically includes an antiplatelet agent and control of cardiovascular risk factors, including smoking cessation, blood pressure control and lipid control with a hydroxy-methyl-glutaryl-CoA reductase inhibitor (statin) [60]. Exercise should also be recommended in appropriate patients, but unsupervised exercise is unlikely to be effective [61].

Other than the above-mentioned general measures, entity-specific treatments should be tailored according to specific patient and diagnosis characteristics. Table 5.2 highlights the treatment of various entities that make up NAPAD.

Conclusions

Peripheral artery disease is common and usually straightforward to diagnose. However, an alert clinician will keep in mind the multiple uncommon conditions that may mimic PAD. Prompt recognition of these conditions will dictate appropriate patient management and is likely to result in improved patient outcomes.

References

1 Selvin E, Erlinger TP. Prevalence of and risk factors for peripheral arterial disease in the United States: results from the National Health and Nutrition Examination Survey, 1999–2000. Circulation. 2004; 110: 738–43.

2 Hirsch AT, Criqui MH, Treat-Jacobson D, *et al*. Peripheral arterial disease detection, awareness, and treatment in primary care. JAMA. 2001; 286: 1317–24.

3 Weinberg I, Jaff MR. Nonatherosclerotic arterial disorders of the lower extremities. Circulation. 2012; 126: 213–22.

4 Rana H, Andrews JS, Chacko BG, *et al.* Mortality in patients with premature lower extremity atherosclerosis. J Vasc Surg. 2013; 57: 28–35 (discussion 35–6).

5 di Marzo L, Cavallaro A. Popliteal vascular entrapment. World J Surg. 2005; 29: S43–5.

6 Levien LJ, Veller MG. Popliteal artery entrapment syndrome: more common than previously recognized. J Vasc Surg. 1999; 30: 587–98.

7 Bouhoutsos J, Daskalakis E. Muscular abnormalities affecting the popliteal vessels. Br J Surg. 1981; 68: 501–6.

8 Gibson MH, Mills JG, Johnson GE, Downs AR. Popliteal entrapment syndrome. Ann Surg. 1977; 185: 341–8.

9 Causey MW, Singh N, Miller S, *et al.* Intraoperative duplex and functional popliteal entrapment syndrome: strategy for effective treatment. Ann Vasc Surg. 2010; 24: 556–61.

10 Angeli AA, Angeli DA, Aggeli CA, Mandrekas DP. Chronic lower leg swelling caused by isolated popliteal venous entrapment. J Vasc Surg. 2011; 54: 851–3.

11 Korngold EC, Jaff MR. Unusual causes of intermittent claudication: popliteal artery entrapment syndrome, cystic adventitial disease, fibromuscular dysplasia, and endofibrosis. Curr Treat Options Cardiovasc Med. 2009; 11: 156–66.

12 Akkersdijk WL, de Ruyter JW, Lapham R, *et al.* Colour duplex ultrasonographic imaging and provocation of popliteal artery compression. Eur J Vasc Endovasc Surg. 1995; 10: 342–5.

13 Hai Z, Guangrui S, Yuan Z, *et al.* CT angiography and MRI in patients with popliteal artery entrapment syndrome. Am J Roentgenol. 2008; 191: 1760–6.

14 Shalhub S, Zierler RE, Smith W, *et al.* Vasospasm as a cause for claudication in athletes with external iliac artery endofibrosis. J Vasc Surg. 2013; 58: 105–11.

15 Peach G, Schep G, Palfreeman R, *et al.* Endofibrosis and kinking of the iliac arteries in athletes: a systematic review. Eur J Vasc Endovasc Surg. 2012; 43: 208–17.

16 Maree AO, Ashequl Islam M, Snuderl M, *et al.* External iliac artery endofibrosis in an amateur runner: hemodynamic, angiographic, histopathological evaluation and percutaneous revascularization. Vasc Med. 2007; 12: 203–6.

17 Slovut DP, Olin JW. Fibromuscular dysplasia. N Engl J Med. 2004; 350: 1862–71.

18 Olin JW, Sealove BA. Diagnosis, management, and future developments of fibromuscular dysplasia. J Vasc Surg. 2011; 53: 826–36.e1.

19 Olin JW, Froehlich J, Gu X, *et al.* The United States Registry for Fibromuscular Dysplasia: results in the first 447 patients. Circulation. 2012; 125: 3182–90.

20 Olin JW, Gornik HL, Bacharach JM, *et al.*, American Heart Association Council on Peripheral Vascular Disease, American Heart Association Council on Clinical Cardiology, American Heart Association Council on Cardiopulmonary, Critical Care, Perioperative and Resuscitation, American Heart Association Council on Cardiovascular Disease in the Young, American Heart Association Council on Cardiovascular Radiology and Intervention, American Heart Association Council on Epidemiology and Prevention, American Heart Association Council on Functional Genomics and Translational Biology, American Heart Association Council for High Blood Pressure Research, American Heart Association Council on the Kidney in Cardiovascular Disease, American Heart Association Stroke Council. Fibromuscular dysplasia: state of the science and critical unanswered questions: a scientific statement from the American Heart Association. Circulation. 2014; 129: 1048–78.

21 Das CJ, Neyaz Z, Thapa P, *et al.* Fibromuscular dysplasia of the renal arteries: a radiological review. Int Urol Nephrol. 2007; 39: 233–8.

22 Gowda MS, Loeb AL, Crouse LJ, Kramer PH. Complementary roles of color-flow duplex imaging and intravascular ultrasound in the diagnosis of renal artery fibromuscular dysplasia: should renal arteriography serve as the "gold standard"? J Am Coll Cardiol. 2003; 41: 1305–11.

23 Kalva SP, Somarouthu B, Jaff MR, Wicky S. Segmental arterial mediolysis: clinical and imaging features at presentation and during follow-up. J Vasc Interv Radiol. 2011; 22: 1380–7.

24 Loeys BL, Schwarze U, Holm T, *et al.* Aneurysm syndromes caused by mutations in the TGF-beta receptor. N Engl J Med. 2006; 355: 788–98.

25 Trinquart L, Mounier-Vehier C, Sapoval M, *et al.* Efficacy of revascularization for renal artery stenosis caused by fibromuscular dysplasia: a systematic review and meta-analysis. Hypertension. 2010; 56: 525–32.

26 Motaganahalli RL, Pennell RC, Mantese VA, Westfall SG. Cystic adventitial disease of the popliteal artery. J Am Coll Surg. 2009; 209: 541.

27 Franca M, Pinto J, Machado R, Fernandez GC. Case 157: bilateral adventitial cystic disease of the popliteal artery. Radiology. 2010; 255: 655–60.

28 Cassar K, Engeset J. Cystic adventitial disease: a trap for the unwary. Eur J Vasc Endovasc Surg. 2005; 29: 93–6.

29 Peterson JJ, Kransdorf MJ, Bancroft LW, Murphey MD. Imaging characteristics of cystic adventitial disease of the peripheral arteries: presentation as soft-tissue masses. Am J Roentgenol. 2003; 180: 621–5.

30 Flanigan DP, Burnham SJ, Goodreau JJ, Bergan JJ. Summary of cases of adventitial cystic disease of the popliteal artery. Ann Surg. 1979; 189: 165–75.

31 Chugh KS, Jain S, Sakhuja V, *et al.* Renovascular hypertension due to Takayasu's arteritis among Indian patients. Q J Med. 1992; 85: 833–43.

32 Connolly JE, Wilson SE, Lawrence PL, Fujitani RM. Middle aortic syndrome: distal thoracic and abdominal coarctation, a disorder with multiple etiologies. J Am Coll Surg. 2002; 194: 774–81.

33 Mwipatayi BP, Jeffery PC, Beningfield SJ, *et al.* Takayasu arteritis: clinical features and management: report of 272 cases. ANZ J Surg. 2005; 75: 110–17.

34 Noris M, Daina E, Gamba S, *et al.* Interleukin-6 and RANTES in Takayasu arteritis: a guide for therapeutic decisions? Circulation. 1999; 100: 55–60.

35 Arend WP, Michel BA, Bloch DA, *et al.* The American College of Rheumatology 1990 criteria for the classification of Takayasu arteritis. Arthritis Rheum. 1990; 33: 1129–34.

36 Nicoletti G, Mannarella C, Nigro A, Sacco A, Olivieri I. The "macaroni sign" of Takayasu's arteritis. J Rheumatol. 2009; 36: 2042–3.

37 Buckley A, Southwood T, Culham G, *et al.* The role of ultrasound in evaluation of Takayasu's arteritis. J Rheumatol. 1991; 18: 1073–80.

38 Gotway MB, Araoz PA, Macedo TA, *et al.* Imaging findings in Takayasu's arteritis. Am J Roentgenol. 2005; 184: 1945–50.

39 Blockmans D. PET in vasculitis. Ann NY Acad Sci. 2011; 1228: 64–70.

40 Arnaud L, Haroche J, Malek Z, *et al.* Is (18)F-fluorodeoxyglucose positron emission tomography scanning a reliable way to assess disease activity in Takayasu arteritis? Arthritis Rheum. 2009; 60: 1193–200.

41 Ogino H, Matsuda H, Minatoya K, *et al.* Overview of late outcome of medical and surgical treatment for Takayasu arteritis. Circulation. 2008; 118: 2738–47.

42 Nishimoto N, Nakahara H, Yoshio-Hoshino N, Mima T. Successful treatment of a patient with Takayasu arteritis using a humanized anti-interleukin-6 receptor antibody. Arthritis Rheum. 2008; 58: 1197–200.

43 Lin YJ, Hwang B, Lee PC, *et al.* Mid-aortic syndrome: a case report and review of the literature. Int J Cardiol. 2008; 123: 348–52.

44 Sen PK, Kinare SG, Engineer SD, Parulkar GB. The Middle Aortic Syndrome. Br Heart J. 1963; 25: 610–8.

45 Verma H, Baliga K, George RK, Tripathi RK. Surgical and endovascular treatment of occlusive aortic syndromes. J Cardiovasc Surg (Torino). 2013; 54: 55–69.

46 Uitto J, Bercovitch L, Terry SF, Terry PF. Pseudoxanthoma elasticum: progress in diagnostics and research towards treatment : Summary of the 2010 PXE International Research Meeting. Am J Med Genet A. 2011; 155A: 1517–26.

47 Hornstrup LS, Tybjaerg-Hansen A, Haase CL, *et al.* Heterozygosity for R1141X in ABCC6 and Risk of Ischemic Vascular Disease. Circ Cardiovasc Genet. 2011; 4: 534–41.

48 von Beckerath O, Gaa J, von Mohrenfels CW, von Beckerath N. Images in cardiovascular medicine. Intermittent claudication in a 28-year-old man with pseudoxanthoma elasticum. Circulation. 2008; 118: 102–4.

49 Hiragi T, Yoshikawa J, Okura H, *et al.* Pseudoxanthoma elasticum associated with unstable angina and Leriche syndrome: a case report. J Cardiol. 1995; 26: 43–9.

50 Spinzi G, Strocchi E, Imperiali G, *et al.* Pseudoxanthoma elasticum: a rare cause of gastrointestinal bleeding. Am J Gastroenterol. 1996; 91: 1631–4.

51 Case records of the Massachusetts General Hospital. Weekly clinicopathological exercises. Case 10–1983. Gastrointestinal bleeding with ocular and cutaneous abnormalities. N Engl J Med. 1983; 308: 579–85.

52 Carter DJ, Woodward DA, Vince FP. Arterial surgery in pseudoxanthoma elasticum. Postgrad Med J. 1976; 52: 291–2.

53 Donas KP, Schulte S, Horsch S. Balloon angioplasty in the treatment of vascular lesions in pseudoxanthoma elasticum. J Vasc Interv Radiol. 2007; 18: 457–9.

54 Hislop M, Tierney P, Murray P, O'Brien M, Mahony N. Chronic exertional compartment syndrome: the controversial "fifth" compartment of the leg. Am J Sports Med. 2003; 31: 770–6.

55 Ehsan O, Darwish A, Edmundson C, *et al*. Non-traumatic lower limb vascular complications in endurance athletes. Review of literature. Eur J Vasc Endovasc Surg. 2004; 28: 1–8.

56 Hutchinson M. Chronic exertional compartment syndrome. Br J Sports Med. 2011; 45: 952–3.

57 Andreisek G, White LM, Sussman MS, *et al*. T2*-weighted and arterial spin labeling MRI of calf muscles in healthy volunteers and patients with chronic exertional compartment syndrome: preliminary experience. Am J Roentgenol. 2009; 193: W327–33.

58 Edwards PH, Jr, Wright ML, Hartman JF. A practical approach for the differential diagnosis of chronic leg pain in the athlete. Am J Sports Med. 2005; 33: 1241–9.

59 Anderson JL, Halperin JL, Albert NM, *et al*. Management of patients with peripheral artery disease (compilation of 2005 and 2011 ACCF/AHA guideline recommendations): a report of the American College of Cardiology Foundation/American Heart Association Task Force on Practice Guidelines. Circulation. 2013; 127: 1425–43.

60 Gandhi S, Weinberg I, Margey R, Jaff MR. Comprehensive medical management of peripheral arterial disease. Prog Cardiovasc Dis. 2011; 54: 2–13.

61 Fokkenrood HJ, Bendermacher BL, Lauret GJ, *et al*. Supervised exercise therapy versus non-supervised exercise therapy for intermittent claudication. Cochrane Database Syst Rev. 2013; 8: CD005263.

6

Medical Therapy of Peripheral Artery Disease

Lee Joseph¹ and Esther S. H. Kim²

¹ *University of Iowa, Iowa City, IA, USA*
² *Vanderbilt University Medical Center, Nashville, TN, USA*

Introduction

Medical therapy of peripheral artery disease (PAD) is aimed at alleviation of symptoms, improvement in quality of life, prevention of limb loss, and prevention of cardiovascular (CV) events. As such, the principal components of medical treatment of PAD include atherosclerotic risk factor (RF) management, claudication pharmacotherapy, exercise therapy, and foot care.

Atherosclerotic Risk Factor Management

As detailed in previous chapters, PAD is a disease of high CV morbidity and mortality [1–3]. Patients with PAD are at a three- to sixfold increased risk for CV mortality compared with age-matched individuals without PAD. Coronary artery disease (CAD) and cerebrovascular disease are highly prevalent among patients with PAD, present in up to 60–80% of this population [4–7]. In a large, international study of stable patients with atherothrombosis in a community setting, patients with PAD had higher annual event rates for myocardial infarction (MI), stroke, CV death or hospitalization (event rate, 21%) compared with patients who had CAD or cerebrovascular disease (event rate, 15%) [8]. As such, PAD is a CAD risk equivalent with similar major modifiable RFs, including tobacco use, diabetes mellitus, hypertension, and hyperlipidemia [9]. Medical management of PAD includes blood pressure (BP) control, lipid control, glycemic control, tobacco cessation, and antiplatelet therapy [10–13]. While an analysis of the National Health and Nutrition Examination Survey (NHANES) data from 1999 to 2004 demonstrated that secondary preventive

Peripheral Artery Disease, Second Edition. Edited by Emile R. Mohler and Michael R. Jaff.
© 2017 John Wiley & Sons Ltd. Published 2017 by John Wiley & Sons Ltd.

therapies reduce all-cause mortality by 65% (hazard ratio [HR] = 0.35; 95% CI: 0.20–0.86; P = 0.02) in PAD subjects without CV disease [14], results of the Reduction of Atherothrombosis for Continued Health (REACH) Registry show that patients with PAD have less optimal control of BP, hyperglycemia, total cholesterol and tobacco cessation compared with those with CAD or cerebrovascular disease ($P < 0.001$) [15].

Hypertension

The Heart Outcomes Prevention Evaluation (HOPE) study of 9,297 high-risk patients including PAD showed that ramipril, an angiotensin-converting enzyme (ACE) inhibitor, significantly reduced the rates of death, MI, and stroke (relative risk = 0.78; 95% CI: 0.70–0.86; $P < 0.001$) independent of antihypertensive effect [16]. Subsequently, in patients with vascular disease or high-risk diabetes, telmisartan, an angiotensin receptor blocker (ARB), was equivalent to ramipril in reducing the risk of CV death, MI, stroke, or hospitalization for heart failure and was associated with less angioedema [17]. Based on the Appropriate Blood Pressure Control in Diabetes (ABCD) study of 950 subjects with type 2 diabetes followed for 5 years, intensive BP lowering to a mean of 128/75 mmHg with enalapril or nisoldipine significantly reduced CV events in PAD patients with diabetes [18]. However, in a study of 4,733 participants with type 2 diabetes, intensive antihypertensive therapy (goal systolic pressure < 120 mmHg), as compared with standard therapy (goal systolic pressure < 140 mmHg) did not markedly reduce the rates of composite outcome of fatal and non-fatal major CV events [19]. It should be noted that PAD, although presumed to be present, was not identified as a subgroup in this study. The significant reduction in the annual stroke rate with intensive BP lowering in this study was also offset by a significant increase in serious antihypertensive treatment-related adverse events. While there have been concerns that beta-blockers could worsen intermittent claudication, a meta-analysis of published randomized controlled trials (RCTs) concluded that beta-blockers do not adversely affect walking capacity or symptoms of intermittent claudication in patients with mild-to-moderate PAD and are safe in such patients [20]. Given the risk of concomitant CAD, beta-blockers should not be withheld if otherwise indicated.

A BP goal of < 140/90 mmHg for PAD patients without diabetes or < 130/80 mmHg for PAD patients with diabetes and chronic renal disease is recommended and the use of ACE inhibitors or ARB is suggested to reduce CV events by the 2013 and 2016 report of the American College of Cardiology Foundation/American Heart Association (ACCF/AHA) Task Force on Practice Guidelines for management of PAD [10, 12, 13]. The eighth Joint National Committee (JNC 8) 2014 evidence-based guidelines for the management of high BP in adults have some major differences from the previously existing guidelines [21]. The JNC 8 report recommends a BP goal of < 150/90 mmHg for persons aged ≥ 60 years, and a BP of < 140/90 mmHg for persons < 59 years old. These authors do not make specific recommendations regarding BP goal and treatment in patients with established atherosclerosis. Initial drug choice for BP control includes an ACE inhibitor, ARB, calcium channel blocker, or thiazide-type diuretic in all subjects except for those who are black and those with chronic kidney disease (CKD). In the black hypertensive population, a calcium channel blocker or thiazide-type diuretic is recommended as initial therapy. In hypertensive persons with CKD, an ACE inhibitor or ARB is recommended as initial or add-on antihypertensive therapy.

Diabetes Mellitus

There is strong epidemiological evidence that favors the association of chronic hyperglycemia with the development of microvascular as well as macrovascular disease in diabetic patients [22–27]. In a meta-analysis of 13 observational studies on glycosylated hemoglobin and CV disease in diabetes mellitus, for a 1% increase in glycosylated hemoglobin level, the pooled relative risks for CV disease were 1.18 (95% CI: 1.10–1.26) in persons with type 2 diabetes and 1.15 (95% CI: 0.92–1.43) in persons with type 1 diabetes [24]. Despite the results of observational data, no RCTs have demonstrated that intensive glycemic control in type 2 diabetes is associated with a significant reduction in macrovascular complications. Intensive blood glucose control substantially decreased the risk of microvascular complications, but not macrovascular complications in the United Kingdom Prospective Diabetes Study of 3,867 patients with type 2 diabetes [28]. Data from Action to Control Cardiovascular Risk in Diabetes (ACCORD) study showed an increase in total and CV disease-related mortality, increased weight gain, and high risk for severe hypoglycemia with intensive glycemic control [29]. There was no significant effect of the type of glucose control on major macrovascular events, CV death, or all-cause death in the Action in Diabetes and Vascular Disease study of 11,140 type 2 diabetics [30]. In the Veterans Affairs Diabetes Trial of 1,791 military veterans with poorly controlled type 2 diabetes, intensive glycemic control had no significant effect on the rates of major CV events or death [31]. In the Diabetes Control and Complications Trial of 1,441 patients with type 1 diabetes, intensive insulin treatment was associated with a 42% non-statistically significant reduction in the risk of the development of macrovascular complications, including PAD, compared with conventional insulin therapy [32]. A 2009 consensus statement of the American Diabetes Association and the European Association for the Study of Diabetes recommended an A1C goal of < 7% for most non-pregnant adults with type 2 diabetes based on practicality and the projected reduction in complications in trials [33]. The 2013 ACCF/AHA PAD guidelines recommend the same A1C goal to reduce microvascular complications and prevent

CV events in PAD patients with diabetes [10]. Based on the 2016 ACCF/AHA PAD guidelines, glycemic control is reasonable to reduce major adverse limb-related outcomes in patients with critical limb ischemia (CLI) [12, 13, 34, 35].

Hyperlipidemia

In patients with PAD, statin therapy not only reduces the incidence of CV events, but also improves PAD symptoms and graft patency. A large prospective observational cohort study of 2,420 consecutive patients with PAD (ankle–brachial index [ABI] ≤ 0.90) found that statin therapy was associated with reduced risk of long-term mortality (HR = 0.46, 95% CI: 0.36–0.58) [36]. In a *post hoc* analysis of the Scandinavian Simvastatin Survival Study (4S), simvastatin achieved a 38% reduction in the risk for new or worsening intermittent claudication ($P = 0.008$) when compared with placebo [37]. There was improvement in mean pain-free walking time after 12 months of treatment for the atorvastatin 80 mg group compared with placebo (63% vs. 38%, respectively; $P = 0.025$) in a randomized, double-blind trial of 354 persons with claudication attributable to PAD [38]. A retrospective analysis of 172 patients showed statin therapy improved graft patency after infra-inguinal bypass grafting with saphenous vein [39]. Statin therapy for all patients with PAD is recommended by the 2016 report of ACCF/AHA PAD management guidelines [13]. The 2013 ACC/AHA guideline on the treatment of blood cholesterol does not identify a particular low-density lipoprotein (LDL) cholesterol goal for statin therapy [40]. Instead, they recommend high-intensity statin therapy in adults with known CV disease who are ≤ 75 years old, while for those > 75 years the benefits and risks of statin therapy need to be assessed.

The clinical benefit of non-statins such as fibric acid derivatives and niacin is not established in PAD patients. The AIM-HIGH investigators showed that niacin did not achieve incremental clinical benefit in patients with atherosclerotic CV disease receiving intensive statin therapy [41]. In patients with type 2 diabetes mellitus at high risk for CV disease, the ACCORD study group found no significant reduction in CV events with the combination of fenofibrate and simvastatin, as compared with simvastatin alone [42]. While the 2013 report of ACCF/AHA PAD management guidelines suggest that treatment with a fibric acid derivative for patients with PAD and low high-density lipoprotein cholesterol, normal LDL cholesterol, and elevated triglycerides, the 2013 ACC/AHA blood cholesterol treatment guideline did not support the routine use of non-statins combined with statin and limits their use for treating statin-intolerant patients or high-risk patients with less than desired response to statins [10, 40].

Tobacco Cessation

The leading RF for incidence and progression of PAD is tobacco use. A meta-analysis of four prospective and 13 cross-sectional studies found a 2.3-fold greater prevalence of symptomatic PAD in current smokers compared with non-smokers [43]. No prospective RCTs have assessed the effect of smoking cessation on CV events in PAD subjects. The Factores de Riesgo y Enfermedad Arterial (FRENA) Registry from Spain evaluated the mortality benefits of smoking cessation in 1,182 current smokers (40% had CAD; 20% had cerebro-vascular disease, and 40% had PAD) [44]. These authors reported that smoking cessation was associated with a significant decrease in mortality in patients with CAD and a non-significant decrease in those with cerebrovascular disease. Other smaller observational studies have reported lower rates of mortality, CV events and limb loss, improved pain-free and total walking distance outcomes and higher rates of open surgical bypass graft patency in individuals with PAD who stopped smoking compared with those who continued to smoke [45–48]. Thromboangiitis obliterans (TAO; Buerger's disease), a non-athero-sclerotic, segmental, inflammatory disease involving small to medium-sized arteries and veins of the extremities, has a strong association with the use of tobacco products. Smoking cessation is crucial to prevent amputation in individuals with TAO.

Interventions for tobacco dependence include behavioral therapy and short-term anti-tobacco dependence pharmacotherapy. The ACCF/AHA guidelines for the management of patients with PAD, and the 2007 TASC II consensus document on the management of PAD guidelines recommend smoking cessation utilizing pharmacological and behavioral treatment strategies for PAD patients who smoke [10, 11, 13]. First-line pharmacotherapeutic options for smoking cessation include varenicline, bupropion, and nicotine replacement therapy (NRT). A Cochrane network meta-analysis of 101,804 patients found that varenicline (smoking cessation rate = 27. 6%) and combination NRT (smoking cessation rate = 31.5%) were the most efficacious pharmacotherapies for achieving continuous or prolonged abstinence at least 6 months from the start of treatment [49].

Clinicians should be aware that both varenicline and bupropion carry a boxed warning on the risk of serious neuropsychiatric events, including depression, suicidal thoughts, and suicide, when taking these drugs. There is also some controversy that varenicline may paradoxically the increase of CV events in those prescribed the medication. A meta-analysis of 14 double-blind RCTs involving 8,216 participants found that varenicline significantly increased the risk of serious adverse CV events compared with placebo [50]. Despite the small magnitude of adverse CV events with varenicline, in relation to its efficacy for smoking cessation, the United States Food and Drug Administration (FDA) suggested that a thorough consideration of its risks and benefits should be made when opting for using varenicline in patients with CV disease.

Electronic cigarettes are gaining popularity among the general population as potential smoking cessation aids. There are limited data regarding the safety and efficacy of electronic cigarettes for smoking cessation, particularly regarding the potential for addiction and inhalation of toxic chemicals. Given these safety concerns, the FDA has not yet approved the use of electronic cigarettes for smoking cessation.

Antiplatelet Agents

The 2002 Antithrombotic Trialists' Collaboration meta-analysis showed a 23% relative risk reduction ($P < 0.004$) in CV events with antiplatelet therapy among symptomatic PAD patients; however, it consisted of trials with heterogeneous antiplatelet regimens and enrollment criteria [51]. The Critical Leg Ischemia Prevention Study (CLIPS) trial of 366 outpatients with stage I–II PAD resulted in a 64% reduction ($P = 0.022$) in the risk of first vascular event (MI, stroke, vascular death) and lower rates of CLI (total, 12 vs. 28; $P = 0.014$) in patients treated with oral aspirin (100 mg daily) compared with placebo [52]. The Prevention of Progression of Arterial Disease and Diabetes (POPADAD) trial, a factorial, multicenter, randomized, double-blind, placebo-controlled Scottish trial, assessed the efficacy of aspirin (100 mg daily) and antioxidants, combined or alone, in comparison with placebo in reducing the development of CV events in 1,276 adults aged ≥ 40 years with type 1 or type 2 diabetes and an ABI ≤ 0.99 but no symptomatic CV disease. There was no evidence of benefit from either aspirin or antioxidant treatment on the composite hierarchical primary end-points of death from coronary heart disease or stroke, non-fatal myocardial infarction or stroke, or amputation above the ankle for CLI [event rate = 18.2% in the aspirin groups vs. 18.3% in the no-aspirin groups, HR (95% CI) = 0.98 (0.76–1.26); event rate = 18.3% in the antioxidant groups vs. 18.2% in the no-antioxidant groups, HR (95% CI) = 1.03 (0.79–1.33)] [53]. In a 2009 meta-analysis of 18 RCTs involving 5,269 individuals with PAD and including the POPADAD trial, aspirin therapy alone or in combination with dipyridamole showed no significant decrease in the primary end-point of CV events (non-fatal MI, non-fatal stroke, and CV death) and a significant reduction in non-fatal stroke [54]. The Aspirin for Asymptomatic Atherosclerosis trial found no statistically significant difference in the risk for vascular events between the aspirin therapy group (100 mg) and the placebo group (HR = 1.03; 95% CI: 0.84–1.27) among 3,350 asymptomatic subjects with a low ABI (≤ 0.95) [55]. The Warfarin Antiplatelet Vascular Evaluation trial concluded that combination of oral anticoagulation therapy and antiplatelet therapy did not significantly reduce CV events among patients with PAD and was associated with an increase in life-threatening bleeding [56].

Clopidogrel 75 mg/day is an alternative to aspirin therapy [10]. A randomized, blinded, trial (CAPRIE) of clopidogrel versus aspirin in 19,185 patients at risk of ischemic events showed a statistically significant ($P = 0.043$) relative risk reduction of 8.7% in the major CV events (combination of ischemic stroke, MI, or vascular death) in favor of clopidogrel (95% CI: 0.3–16.5) [57]. The 2016 ACCF/

AHA PAD guideline writing committee recommended aspirin 75–325 mg/day or clopidogrel 75 mg/day for secondary prevention in patients with symptomatic PAD, and suggested antiplatelet therapy in patients with asymptomatic PAD [13]. A *post hoc* analysis of the 3,096 patients with PAD from the CHARISMA trial provided evidence that clopidogrel plus aspirin was more effective than aspirin alone in preventing MI (HR = 0.63; 95% CI: 0.42–0.96; P = 0.029) and hospitalization for ischemic events (HR = 0.81; 95% CI: 0.68–0.95; P = 0.011), although there was an increase in minor bleeding (odds ratio = 1.99; 95% CI: 1.69–2.34; P < 0.001) [58]. The combination of aspirin and clopidogrel may be considered in symptomatic PAD patients without significant bleeding risk after lower extremity revascularization.[13]

Patients with aspirin or clopidogrel resistance pose a challenge in some patients with PAD, and newer antiplatelet agents may provide alternate choices. Prasugrel is an effective alternative to clopidogrel, although there is an increased bleeding risk in patients undergoing percutaneous coronary intervention (PCI) [59]. The data on efficacy and safety of prasugrel for secondary prevention of PAD patients not undergoing PCI are not yet available. The novel P2Y12 antagonist, ticagrelor, improved peripheral endothelial function after forearm ischemia compared with no adenosine diphosphate blocker, clopidogrel, or prasugrel treatment (P < 0.01) [60]. In a randomized, double-blind, placebo-controlled trial in 3,787 patients with a history of claudication and an ABI < 0.85 or prior revascularization for limb ischemia, vorapaxar, a novel protease-activated receptor-1 antagonist, had no significant reduction in the risk of CV death, MI, or stroke; however, voraxapar significantly reduced the rates of hospitalization for acute limb ischemia (2.3% vs. 3.9%; HR = 0.58; 95% CI: 0.39–0.86; P = 0.006) and peripheral artery revascularization (18.4% vs. 22.2%; HR = 0.84; 95% CI: 0.73–0.97; P = 0.017) [61]. There was an increased risk of bleeding with vorapaxar versus placebo (7.4% vs. 4.5%; HR = 1.62; 95% CI: 1.21–2.18; P = 0.001). The FDA approved vorapaxar for patients with PAD. Evidence on the role of these newer antiplatelet agents in PAD continues to emerge, but as per the 2016 ACCF/AHA PAD guidelines, the overall benefit of adding voraxapar to existing antiplatelet therapy for symptomatic PAD is unknown [13].

Management of Claudication

Strategies to improve claudication symptoms include pharmacological drugs, PAD exercise rehabilitation therapy, and revascularization. The claudication pharmacotherapy and exercise therapy are detailed here; discussion on the revascularization strategy can be found in the chapters on endovascular and surgical treatment of PAD.

Claudication Pharmacotherapy

Two FDA-approved drugs for claudication therapy are cilostazol and pentoxifylline; however, only cilostazol is recommended by the 2016 ACCF/AHA PAD guidelines [13].

Cilostazol

Cilostazol is a phosphodiesterase type III inhibitor leading to an increase in intracellular cyclic adenosine monophosphate (cAMP) levels. It inhibits platelet aggregation and causes weak vasodilation. In addition to its antiplatelet and vasodilator effect, it is an inhibitor of smooth muscle cell proliferation and intimal hyperplasia, a favorable modifier of plasma lipoproteins and results in modest improvements in ABI at rest and after exercise [62–64]. However, the mechanism of effect of cilostazol in PAD is not well established. Cilostazol, compared with placebo, improved both pain-free and maximal treadmill walking distance in four randomized, placebo-controlled trials comprising 1,534 patients, and was superior to pentoxifylline in one trial [64–67]. Cilostazol may also reduce the restenosis risk after endovascular therapy in patients with femoro-popliteal PAD [68]. In the absence of contraindications, a trial of cilostazol (100 mg orally two times per day) is indicated in patients with lower extremity PAD and intermittent claudication for improving symptoms and walking distance [10, 13]. Although some patients may experience clinical improvement as early as 2–4 weeks after initiation of cilostazol, a 3-month minimum trial period should be given for this drug [69]. Most common side-effects of this drug are headache, diarrhea, palpitations, and dizziness. Because of the increase in mortality associated with milrinone (another type 3 phosphodiesterase inhibitor) in heart failure patients, cilostazol use is contraindicated in patients with heart failure.

Exercise Therapy

For patients with claudication, a supervised exercise training program for a minimum of 30–45 minutes, in sessions performed at least three times per week for a minimum of 12 weeks is recommended [10, 13]. The salient features of supervised exercise therapy are summarized in Box 6.1. Exercise training for claudication improves endothelial function, muscle metabolism and hemorrheology, reduces inflammation, and possibly promotes vascular angiogenesis [70]. In an RCT involving 156 patients with PAD, supervised treadmill exercise improved 6-minute walk performance, treadmill walking performance, brachial artery flow-mediated dilation, and quality of life of PAD participants with and without claudication [71]. A meta-analysis of 21 studies showed that the pain-free walking distance increased by 179% ($P < 0.001$), and the maximal walking distance

---

Box 6.1 Salient features of claudication exercise rehabilitation program [10, 70]

- One-to-one supervision by an exercise physiologist, physical therapist, or nurse
- A minimum of three sessions/week for > 3 months
- Each session lasts 45–60 minutes (initially 35 minutes of intermittent walking; increased by 5 minutes until 50 minutes of intermittent walking can be accomplished along with 5–10 minutes of warm-up and cool-down sessions)
- Using motorized treadmill or a track
- Monitor claudication threshold and cardiovascular status
- Uncertain optimal exercise regimen and intensity

---

increased by 122% ($P < 0.001$) with a program for exercise rehabilitation [72]. Such programs are highly cost-effective when compared with catheter-based revascularization [73]. Unfortunately, lack of reimbursement for a supervised exercise program is a major limiting factor in its widespread utilization. A structured community- or home-based exercise program with behavioral change techniques can be beneficial [13]. The efficacy of unstructured exercise programs is not well established. A supervised exercise program showed a statistically significant benefit on treadmill walking distance (maximal and pain-free) compared with non-supervised regimens in a meta-analysis of 14 studies involving a total of 1,002 participants with PAD [74]. A recent trial demonstrated that both a home-based exercise program, quantified with a step activity monitor, and a standard supervised exercise program showed similar adherence and efficacy in improving claudication measures [75].

Claudication Management Strategies: A Comparison

Several studies have evaluated the comparative efficacy of medical therapy and revascularization for PAD management. The CLEVER trial studied 111 patients with aortoiliac PAD [76]. It is the largest multicenter RCT to date comparing revascularization, supervised exercise rehabilitation and optimal medical care (OMC; CV risk reduction plus cilostazol). The three treatment arms consisted of OMC alone, OMC plus supervised exercise rehabilitation (three times a week for 26 weeks), and OMC plus stenting revascularization. A fourth arm of OMC plus endovascular revascularization and supervised exercise rehabilitation was removed due to the relatively low enrollment. The primary end-point was maximal treadmill walking time at 6 and 18 months' follow-up. Secondary end-points included claudication onset time, community-based walking by pedometer, quality of life questionnaires (WIQ, Peripheral Artery Questionnaire, Medical

Outcomes Study 12-Item Short Form) and atherosclerosis biomarkers. Both supervised exercise and stenting showed significant beneficial effects over OMC at 6 months. Supervised exercise resulted in significantly superior treadmill performance compared with OMC and stenting arms. Stenting resulted in a better self-reported quality of life compared with OMC and supervised exercise arms, although the supervised exercise arm also showed significant improvement in quality of life compared with OMC. The mechanisms of treatment benefit and optimal outcome measures for claudication trials remain unanswered. This study and others support the initial treatment of claudication with a supervised exercise program. It also raises the question of whether cilostazol is ineffective in aortoiliac PAD.

Lower Extremity Wound Care

Critical limb ischemia occurs in 1–2% of patients with PAD older than 50 years over a 5-year period [77]. In a patient with PAD, especially those with diabetes mellitus, self-foot examination, healthy foot behaviors, prompt diagnosis and treatment of foot infection using an interdisciplinary approach, and biannual foot examination by a clinician are critical to prevent CLI [13]. Patients with CLI can present with rest pain or tissue loss (ulceration or gangrene). CLI will lead to amputation if aggressive wound care and adequate perfusion are not achieved.

The principal components of wound care include a thorough evaluation of the underlying etiology, maintaining adequate perfusion, wound bed preparation, moist wound healing, control of edema, infection control, offloading and appropriate systemic disease control [78]. A well-structured wound care plan requires a multidisciplinary approach involving wound care specialists and nurses, podiatrists, vascular specialists, plastic surgeons, prosthetists and orthotists.

Every patient with a lower extremity wound should undergo careful assessment to exclude other causes of ulceration, including neoplastic, metabolic, inflammatory, infectious, and traumatic processes. A thorough assessment for infection and control of the infection, if present, are fundamental components of wound management. Although unusual, lower extremity edema may coexist in patients with ischemic lower extremity ulceration and can impair wound healing. Evaluation of the underlying cause of the edema is critical in determining the appropriate strategies to address this problem. Wound care in patients with coexistent ischemic leg and chronic venous insufficiency is particularly challenging, and caution should be applied when using standard approaches for edema management, such as compression therapy, leg elevation, and calf muscle pump exercises. Mechanical offloading options range from crutches or walkers to customized orthotics and prosthetic devices. Such options must be considered for each patient, and may require involvement of a prosthetist and/or orthotist.

Wound bed preparation involves debridement using one of the following modalities: surgical, mechanical, enzymatic, autolytic, and bio-surgical. In patients who are yet to be revascularized, aggressive surgical debridement should be avoided. Autolytic debridement can worsen infection and must therefore be avoided in the setting of active infection. A topical wound dressing that maintains appropriate moisture balance must be selected to promote adequate wound healing. Tight glycemic control, adequate nutritional status, smoking cessation and optimal levels of hemoglobin and vitamins are important to achieve wound healing [79]. Wounds that fail to improve despite standard care may require advanced care with topical growth factors, negative pressure wound therapy, and/or bioengineered alternative tissues.

Summary

In conclusion, every PAD patient should receive aggressive secondary prevention measures to reduce CV events using contemporary guideline-based strategies for BP control, lipid control, glycemic control, tobacco cessation, and antiplatelet therapy. Pharmacotherapy, exercise therapy, and revascularization are the options to manage claudication. Cilostazol is the preferred agent for treating claudication in the absence of contraindications. While a supervised exercise training program is recommended for patients with claudication, the efficacy of unstructured exercise therapy for this purpose is not well established. Aggressive wound care with a multidisciplinary approach is crucial in preventing limb loss in PAD patients with lower extremity wounds.

References

1 Howell MA, Colgan MP, Seeger RW, *et al.* Relationship of severity of lower limb peripheral vascular disease to mortality and morbidity: a six-year follow-up study. J Vasc Surg. 1989; 9(5): 691–6; discussion 6–7.
2 Criqui MH, Langer RD, Fronek A, *et al.* Mortality over a period of 10 years in patients with peripheral arterial disease. N Engl J Med. 1992; 326(6): 381–6.
3 McKenna M, Wolfson S, Kuller L. The ratio of ankle and arm arterial pressure as an independent predictor of mortality. Atherosclerosis. 1991; 87(2–3): 119–28.
4 Valentine RJ, Grayburn PA, Eichhorn EJ, *et al.* Coronary artery disease is highly prevalent among patients with premature peripheral vascular disease. J Vasc Surg. 1994; 19(4): 668–74.

5 McFalls EO, Ward HB, Moritz TE, *et al.* Coronary-artery revascularization before elective major vascular surgery. N Engl J Med. 2004; 351(27): 2795–804.

6 Klop RB, Eikelboom BC, Taks AC. Screening of the internal carotid arteries in patients with peripheral vascular disease by colour-flow duplex scanning. Eur J Vasc Surg. 1991; 5(1): 41–5.

7 Cheng SW, Wu LL, Ting AC, *et al.* Screening for asymptomatic carotid stenosis in patients with peripheral vascular disease: a prospective study and risk factor analysis. Cardiovasc Surg. 1999; 7(3): 303–9.

8 Steg PG, Bhatt DL, Wilson PW, *et al.* One-year cardiovascular event rates in outpatients with atherothrombosis. JAMA. 2007; 297(11): 1197–206.

9 Fowkes FG, Rudan D, Rudan I, *et al.* Comparison of global estimates of prevalence and risk factors for peripheral artery disease in 2000 and 2010: a systematic review and analysis. Lancet. 2013; 382(9901): 1329–40.

10 Anderson JL, Halperin JL, Albert NM, *et al.* Management of patients with peripheral artery disease (compilation of 2005 and 2011 ACCF/AHA guideline recommendations): a report of the American College of Cardiology Foundation/American Heart Association Task Force on Practice Guidelines. Circulation. 2013; 127(13): 1425–43.

11 Norgren L, Hiatt WR, Dormandy JA, *et al.* Inter-Society Consensus for the Management of Peripheral Arterial Disease (TASC II). Eur J Vasc Endovasc Surg. 2007; 33 Suppl 1: S1–75.

12 Gerhard-Herman MD, Gornik HL, *et al.* 2016 AHA/ACC Guideline on the Management of Patients With Lower Extremity Peripheral Artery Disease: Executive Summary: A Report of the American College of Cardiology/ American Heart Association Task Force on Clinical Practice Guidelines. Circulation. 2017; 135(12): e686–e725.

13 Gerhard-Herman MD, Gornik HL, Barrett C, *et al.* 2016 AHA/ACC Guideline on the Management of Patients With Lower Extremity Peripheral Artery Disease: A Report of the American College of Cardiology/American Heart Association Task Force on Clinical Practice Guidelines. J Am Coll Cardiol. 2017; 69(11): e71–e126.

14 Pande RL, Perlstein TS, Beckman JA, Creager MA. Secondary prevention and mortality in peripheral artery disease: National Health and Nutrition Examination Study, 1999 to 2004. Circulation. 2011; 124(1): 17–23.

15 Cacoub PP, Abola MT, Baumgartner I, *et al.* Cardiovascular risk factor control and outcomes in peripheral artery disease patients in the Reduction of Atherothrombosis for Continued Health (REACH) Registry. Atherosclerosis. 2009; 204(2): e86–92.

16 Yusuf S, Sleight P, Pogue J, *et al.* Effects of an angiotensin-converting-enzyme inhibitor, ramipril, on cardiovascular events in high-risk patients. The Heart Outcomes Prevention Evaluation Study Investigators. N Engl J Med. 2000; 342(3): 145–53.

17 Yusuf S, Teo KK, Pogue J, *et al.* Telmisartan, ramipril, or both in patients at high risk for vascular events. N Engl J Med. 2008; 358(15): 1547–59.

18 Mehler PS, Coll JR, Estacio R, *et al.* Intensive blood pressure control reduces the risk of cardiovascular events in patients with peripheral arterial disease and type 2 diabetes. Circulation. 2003; 107(5): 753–6.

19 Cushman WC, Evans GW, Byington RP, *et al.* Effects of intensive blood-pressure control in type 2 diabetes mellitus. N Engl J Med. 2010; 362(17): 1575–85.

20 Radack K, Deck C. Beta-adrenergic blocker therapy does not worsen intermittent claudication in subjects with peripheral arterial disease. A meta-analysis of randomized controlled trials. Arch Intern Med. 1991; 151(9): 1769–76.

21 James PA, Oparil S, Carter BL, *et al.* 2014 evidence-based guideline for the management of high blood pressure in adults: report from the panel members appointed to the Eighth Joint National Committee (JNC 8). JAMA. 2014; 311(5): 507–20.

22 Khaw KT, Wareham N, Bingham S, *et al.* Association of hemoglobin A1c with cardiovascular disease and mortality in adults: the European prospective investigation into cancer in Norfolk. Ann Intern Med. 2004; 141(6): 413–20.

23 Kuusisto J, Mykkanen L, Pyorala K, Laakso M. NIDDM and its metabolic control predict coronary heart disease in elderly subjects. Diabetes. 1994; 43(8): 960–7.

24 Selvin E, Marinopoulos S, Berkenblit G, *et al.* Meta-analysis: glycosylated hemoglobin and cardiovascular disease in diabetes mellitus. Ann Intern Med. 2004; 141(6): 421–31.

25 Selvin E, Steffes MW, Zhu H, *et al.* Glycated hemoglobin, diabetes, and cardiovascular risk in nondiabetic adults. N Engl J Med. 2010; 362(9): 800–11.

26 Selvin E, Coresh J, Golden SH, *et al.* Glycemic control, atherosclerosis, and risk factors for cardiovascular disease in individuals with diabetes: the atherosclerosis risk in communities study. Diabetes Care. 2005; 28(8): 1965–73.

27 Meigs JB, Singer DE, Sullivan LM, *et al.* Metabolic control and prevalent cardiovascular disease in non-insulin-dependent diabetes mellitus (NIDDM): The NIDDM Patient Outcome Research Team. Am J Med. 1997; 102(1): 38–47.

28 UK Prospective Diabetes Study (UKPDS) Group. Intensive blood-glucose control with sulphonylureas or insulin compared with conventional treatment and risk of complications in patients with type 2 diabetes (UKPDS 33). Lancet. 1998; 352(9131): 837–53.

29 Ismail-Beigi F, Craven T, Banerji MA, *et al.* Effect of intensive treatment of hyperglycaemia on microvascular outcomes in type 2 diabetes: an analysis of the ACCORD randomised trial. Lancet. 2010; 376(9739): 419–30.

30 Patel A, MacMahon S, Chalmers J, *et al.* Intensive blood glucose control and vascular outcomes in patients with type 2 diabetes. N Engl J Med. 2008; 358(24): 2560–72.

31 Duckworth W, Abraira C, Moritz T, *et al.* Glucose control and vascular complications in veterans with type 2 diabetes. N Engl J Med. 2009; 360(2): 129–39.

32 Effect of intensive diabetes management on macrovascular events and risk factors in the Diabetes Control and Complications Trial. Am J Cardiol. 1995; 75(14): 894–903.

33 Nathan DM, Buse JB, Davidson MB, *et al.* Medical management of hyperglycemia in type 2 diabetes: a consensus algorithm for the initiation and adjustment of therapy: a consensus statement of the American Diabetes Association and the European Association for the Study of Diabetes. Diabetes Care. 2009; 32(1): 193–203.

34 Singh S, Armstrong EJ, Sherif W, *et al.* Association of elevated fasting glucose with lower patency and increased major adverse limb events among patients with diabetes undergoing infrapopliteal balloon angioplasty. Vasc Med. 2014; 19(4): 307–14.

35 Takahara M, Kaneto H, Iida O, *et al.* The influence of glycemic control on the prognosis of Japanese patients undergoing percutaneous transluminal angioplasty for critical limb ischemia. Diabetes Care. 2010; 33(12): 2538–42.

36 Feringa HH, van Waning VH, Bax JJ, *et al.* Cardioprotective medication is associated with improved survival in patients with peripheral arterial disease. J Am Coll Cardiol. 2006; 47(6): 1182–7.

37 Pedersen TR, Kjekshus J, Pyorala K, *et al.* Effect of simvastatin on ischemic signs and symptoms in the Scandinavian simvastatin survival study (4S). Am J Cardiol. 1998; 81(3): 333–5.

38 Mohler ER, 3rd, Hiatt WR, Creager MA. Cholesterol reduction with atorvastatin improves walking distance in patients with peripheral arterial disease. Circulation. 2003; 108(12): 1481–6.

39 Abbruzzese TA, Havens J, Belkin M, *et al.* Statin therapy is associated with improved patency of autogenous infrainguinal bypass grafts. J Vasc Surg. 2004; 39(6): 1178–85.

40 Stone NJ, Robinson J, Lichtenstein AH, *et al.* 2013 ACC/AHA Guideline on the Treatment of Blood Cholesterol to Reduce Atherosclerotic Cardiovascular Risk in Adults: A Report of the American College of Cardiology/American Heart Association Task Force on Practice Guidelines. Circulation. 2013.

41 Boden WE, Probstfield JL, Anderson T, *et al.* Niacin in patients with low HDL cholesterol levels receiving intensive statin therapy. N Engl J Med. 2011; 365(24): 2255–67.

42 Ginsberg HN, Elam MB, Lovato LC, *et al.* Effects of combination lipid therapy in type 2 diabetes mellitus. N Engl J Med. 2010; 362(17): 1563–74.

43 Willigendael EM, Teijink JA, Bartelink ML, *et al.* Influence of smoking on incidence and prevalence of peripheral arterial disease. J Vasc Surg. 2004; 40(6): 1158–65.

44 Alvarez LR, Balibrea JM, Surinach JM, *et al.* Smoking cessation and outcome in stable outpatients with coronary, cerebrovascular, or peripheral artery disease. Eur J Prev Cardiol. 2013; 20(3): 486–95.

45 Ameli FM, Stein M, Provan JL, Prosser R. The effect of postoperative smoking on femoropopliteal bypass grafts. Ann Vasc Surg. 1989; 3(1): 20–5.

46 Quick CR, Cotton LT. The measured effect of stopping smoking on intermittent claudication. Br J Surg. 1982; 69 Suppl: S24–6.

47 Jonason T, Bergstrom R. Cessation of smoking in patients with intermittent claudication. Effects on the risk of peripheral vascular complications, myocardial infarction and mortality. Acta Med Scand. 1987; 221(3): 253–60.

48 Girolami B, Bernardi E, Prins MH, *et al.* Treatment of intermittent claudication with physical training, smoking cessation, pentoxifylline, or nafronyl: a meta-analysis. Arch Intern Med. 1999; 159(4): 337–45.

49 Cahill K, Stevens S, Perera R, Lancaster T. Pharmacological interventions for smoking cessation: an overview and network meta-analysis. Cochrane Database Syst Rev. 2013; 5: CD009329.

50 Singh S, Loke YK, Spangler JG, Furberg CD. Risk of serious adverse cardiovascular events associated with varenicline: a systematic review and meta-analysis. CMAJ. 2011; 183(12): 1359–66.

51 Collaborative meta-analysis of randomised trials of antiplatelet therapy for prevention of death, myocardial infarction, and stroke in high risk patients. BMJ. 2002; 324(7329): 71–86.

52 Catalano M, Born G, Peto R. Prevention of serious vascular events by aspirin amongst patients with peripheral arterial disease: randomized, double-blind trial. J Intern Med. 2007; 261(3): 276–84.

53 Belch J, MacCuish A, Campbell I, *et al.* The prevention of progression of arterial disease and diabetes (POPADAD) trial: factorial randomised placebo controlled trial of aspirin and antioxidants in patients with diabetes and asymptomatic peripheral arterial disease. BMJ. 2008; 337: a1840.

54 Berger JS, Krantz MJ, Kittelson JM, Hiatt WR. Aspirin for the prevention of cardiovascular events in patients with peripheral artery disease: a meta-analysis of randomized trials. JAMA. 2009; 301(18): 1909–19.

55 Fowkes FG, Price JF, Stewart MC, *et al.* Aspirin for prevention of cardiovascular events in a general population screened for a low ankle brachial index: a randomized controlled trial. JAMA. 2010; 303(9): 841–8.

56 Anand S, Yusuf S, Xie C, *et al.* Oral anticoagulant and antiplatelet therapy and peripheral arterial disease. N Engl J Med. 2007; 357(3): 217–27.

57 CAPRIE Steering Committee. A randomised, blinded, trial of clopidogrel versus aspirin in patients at risk of ischaemic events (CAPRIE). Lancet. 1996; 348(9038): 1329–39.

58 Cacoub PP, Bhatt DL, Steg PG, *et al.* Patients with peripheral arterial disease in the CHARISMA trial. Eur Heart J. 2009; 30(2): 192–201.

59 Wiviott SD, Braunwald E, McCabe CH, *et al.* Prasugrel versus clopidogrel in patients with acute coronary syndromes. N Engl J Med. 2007; 357(20): 2001–15.

60 Torngren K, Ohman J, Salmi H, *et al.* Ticagrelor improves peripheral arterial function in patients with a previous acute coronary syndrome. Cardiology. 2013; 124(4): 252–8.

61 Bonaca MP, Scirica BM, Creager MA, *et al.* Vorapaxar in patients with peripheral artery disease: results from TRA2°P-TIMI 50. Circulation. 2013; 127(14): 1522–9, 1529e1–6.

62 Mohler ER, 3rd, Beebe HG, Salles-Cuhna S, *et al.* Effects of cilostazol on resting ankle pressures and exercise-induced ischemia in patients with intermittent claudication. Vasc Med. 2001; 6(3): 151–6.

63 Elam MB, Heckman J, Crouse JR, *et al.* Effect of the novel antiplatelet agent cilostazol on plasma lipoproteins in patients with intermittent claudication. Arterioscler Thromb Vasc Biol. 1998; 18(12): 1942–7.

64 Money SR, Herd JA, Isaacsohn JL, *et al.* Effect of cilostazol on walking distances in patients with intermittent claudication caused by peripheral vascular disease. J Vasc Surg. 1998; 27(2): 267–74; discussion 74–5.

65 Beebe HG, Dawson DL, Cutler BS, *et al.* A new pharmacological treatment for intermittent claudication: results of a randomized, multicenter trial. Arch Intern Med. 1999; 159(17): 2041–50.

66 Dawson DL, Cutler BS, Hiatt WR, *et al.* A comparison of cilostazol and pentoxifylline for treating intermittent claudication. Am J Med. 2000; 109(7): 523–30.

67 Dawson DL, Cutler BS, Meissner MH, Strandness DE, Jr. Cilostazol has beneficial effects in treatment of intermittent claudication: results from a multicenter, randomized, prospective, double-blind trial. Circulation. 1998; 98(7): 678–86.

68 Iida O, Yokoi H, Soga Y, *et al.* Cilostazol reduces angiographic restenosis after endovascular therapy for femoropopliteal lesions in the Sufficient Treatment of Peripheral Intervention by Cilostazol study. Circulation. 2013; 127(23): 2307–15.

69 Chi YW, Jaff MR. Optimal risk factor modification and medical management of the patient with peripheral arterial disease. Catheter Cardiovasc Interv. 2008; 71(4): 475–89.

70 Stewart KJ, Hiatt WR, Regensteiner JG, Hirsch AT. Exercise training for claudication. N Engl J Med. 2002; 347(24): 1941–51.

71 McDermott MM, Ades P, Guralnik JM, *et al.* Treadmill exercise and resistance training in patients with peripheral arterial disease with and without intermittent claudication: a randomized controlled trial. JAMA. 2009; 301(2): 165–74.

72 Gardner AW, Poehlman ET. Exercise rehabilitation programs for the treatment of claudication pain. A meta-analysis. JAMA. 1995; 274(12): 975–80.

73 Treesak C, Kasemsup V, Treat-Jacobson D, *et al.* Cost-effectiveness of exercise training to improve claudication symptoms in patients with peripheral arterial disease. Vasc Med. 2004; 9(4): 279–85.

74 Fokkenrood HJ, Bendermacher BL, Lauret GJ, *et al.* Supervised exercise therapy versus non-supervised exercise therapy for intermittent claudication. Cochrane Database Syst Rev. 2013; 8: CD005263.

75 Gardner AW, Parker DE, Montgomery PS, *et al.* Efficacy of quantified home-based exercise and supervised exercise in patients with intermittent claudication: a randomized controlled trial. Circulation. 2011; 123(5): 491–8.

76 Murphy TP, Cutlip DE, Regensteiner JG, *et al.* Supervised exercise versus primary stenting for claudication resulting from aortoiliac peripheral artery disease: six-month outcomes from the claudication: exercise versus endoluminal revascularization (CLEVER) study. Circulation. 2012; 125(1): 130–9.

77 Weitz JI, Byrne J, Clagett GP, *et al.* Diagnosis and treatment of chronic arterial insufficiency of the lower extremities: a critical review. Circulation. 1996; 94(11): 3026–49.

78 Bumpus K, Maier MA. The ABC's of wound care. Curr Cardiol Rep. 2013; 15(4): 346.

79 Kavalukas SL, Barbul A. Nutrition and wound healing: an update. Plast Reconstr Surg. 2011; 127 Suppl 1: 38S–43S.

7

Endovascular Treatment of Peripheral Artery Disease

Vikram Prasanna[1], Jay Giri[1] and R. Kevin Rogers[2]

[1] *Cardiovascular Medicine Division, University of Pennsylvania, PA, USA*
[2] *Division of Cardiology, University of Colorado, Aurora, CO, USA*

Introduction

The first lower extremity endovascular procedure was performed by Dotter and Judkins in 1964 [1]. Since that time, the volume of endovascular procedures has increased considerably and is now established as a viable alternative to surgery in patients who have failed supervised exercise and medical therapy. For example, from 1998 to 2003, the national per-capita rate of percutaneous lower extremity arterial revascularization was projected to have increased by 53% [2]. With the increase in operator experience and concomitant technologic advances, procedural success rates are high, though there is a lack of randomized trial data comparing endovascular therapies.

The indications for endovascular treatment of peripheral artery disease (PAD) are to improve walking ability for patients with lifestyle-limiting claudication and to promote limb salvage in patients with critical limb ischemia (CLI; ischemic rest pain and/or tissue loss). These two populations differ substantially in limb prognosis, anatomic complexity, level of anatomic disease, treatment goals, and overall survival. In this chapter, the clinical background, technical considerations, and periprocedural management of endovascular treatment for patients with claudication and CLI are discussed.

Clinical Background

Intermittent Claudication

Claudication is discomfort in a specific group of lower extremity muscles that occurs with exertion and is relieved with rest [3]. Although multiple disorders

Peripheral Artery Disease, Second Edition. Edited by Emile R. Mohler and Michael R. Jaff.
© 2017 John Wiley & Sons Ltd. Published 2017 by John Wiley & Sons Ltd.

Table 7.1 Classification of claudication and critical limb ischemia.

Fontaine		Rutherford		
Stage	Clinical	Grade	Category	Clinical
Claudication				
I	Asymptomatic	0	0	Asymptomatic
IIa	Mild claudication	I	1	Mild claudication
IIb	Moderate to severe claudication	I	2	Moderate claudication
		I	3	Severe claudication
Critical limb ischemia				
III	Ischemic rest pain	II	4	Ischemic rest pain
IV	Ulceration or gangrene	III	5	Minor tissue loss
		III	6	Major tissue loss

can cause claudication, the most common is atherosclerotic PAD. The location of symptoms correlates with the location of hemodynamically significant disease. For example, atherosclerotic occlusion in the aorto-iliac arterial segments can result in complaints of buttock, hip, thigh, or calf discomfort. Calf claudication can result from hemodynamically significant obstruction of any of the arteries cephalad to the calf. Disease of the superficial femoral artery (SFA) in the mid-thigh is a particularly frequent location resulting in calf claudication. Foot claudication may occur from tibioperoneal arterial disease. There are two widely used systems for classification of claudication (Table 7.1).

The clinical significance of claudication is primarily quality of life, rather than threat of limb loss. In patients with PAD and claudication, amputation is a relatively rare outcome, with only 1–2% of claudicants ever requiring major amputation over a 5-year period [4]. Indeed, in one study, 50% of claudicants became symptom-free during 5 years of follow-up [4]. Deterioration is most frequent during the first year after diagnosis (6–9%) compared with 2–3% per year thereafter [4].

Before undergoing an evaluation for revascularization, patients with claudication should have significant functional impairment with a reasonable likelihood of symptomatic improvement and absence of other diseases that would equally limit activity levels (e.g., angina pectoris, congestive heart failure, chronic respiratory diseases, orthopedic limitations). Additionally, optimal medical therapy and supervised exercise programs should be pursued prior to revascularization [5]. Endovascular procedures are indicated for individuals with a vocational or lifestyle disability due to claudication when clinical features suggest a reasonable likelihood of sustainable symptomatic improvement following revascularization, when there has been an inadequate response to exercise or pharmacological therapy and/or when there is a favorable benefit/risk ratio [3].

Critical Limb Ischemia

Limb Prognosis/Overall Survival

In contrast to patients with claudication, those with CLI are at increased risk of limb loss. The natural history of patients with CLI was demonstrated in the TAMIRIS trial, which compared gene therapy with placebo in unrevascularized patients with CLI [6, 7]. In the 266 patients randomized to placebo, the 1-year incidence of amputation was 21% and the mortality rate was 15%.

Typical Anatomy in Patients with CLI

Patients with CLI often have multi-level disease, and the prevalence of disease below the knee is high. In a retrospective report of 450 patients who underwent infrainguinal intervention at two academic institutions, the prevalence of patients who had popliteal or tibioperoneal occlusions was 55% [8]. Of these patients, 65% had an additional occlusion at the aorto-iliac or femoral level [8]. Thus, expertise in below-knee intervention is important for the endovascular specialist treating CLI.

Patency Issues

In contrast to patients with claudication or ischemic rest pain, long-term patency for patients with tissue loss is often less important. The degree of arterial perfusion to heal a wound exceeds the degree of arterial flow necessary to maintain relatively healthy tissue integrity [9]. Thus, the duration of patency is often necessary only to heal a wound in a CLI patient, after which appropriate footwear and wound prevention measures will suffice. For example, in a meta-analysis of 30 observational studies including 2557 patients with CLI who underwent endovascular treatment of tibioperoneal arteries, primary patency at 1 year was only $58.1 \pm 4.6\%$, but limb salvage was $86 \pm 2.7\%$ [10].

Indications for Endovascular Therapy for CLI

The indications for endovascular treatment in patients with CLI are limb salvage with the goal of improved quality of life and limb function [11]. The decision to proceed with percutaneous revascularization is often complex. The likelihood of healing and achieving a functional limb and ambulatory status must be considered, as should a patient's projected survival. The ability to offer meticulous wound care, and the patient's desire to comply with ongoing wound care is paramount. Finally, a patient's clinical risk must be balanced. In addition, in the case of ischemic rest pain, reasonable patency and ongoing surveillance become important. The updated American College of Cardiology Foundation and American Heart Association (ACCF/AHA) guidelines from 2013 for percutaneous revascularization of patients with CLI are summarized in Table 7.2 [12].

Table 7.2 Updated American College of Cardiology Foundation and American Heart Association (ACCF/AHA) Guidelines on endovascular treatment for patients with critical limb ischemia (CLI) [12].

Class	Level of evidence	Summary of recommendation
I	C	Inflow lesions should be treated prior to outflow lesions
I	B	If manifestations of CLI persist after inflow revascularization, outflow revascularization should be pursued
I	C	For angiographically indeterminate inflow lesions, intra-arterial pressure gradients should be assessed with vasodilator administration
IIa	B	If a patient's life expectancy is < 2 years or if autologous venous conduit is not available, percutaneous revascularization is reasonable

Background for Endovascular Therapy

Anatomy

Endovascular interventionalists require special knowledge of peripheral arterial anatomy to obtain the highest quality angiograms, to achieve optimal perfusion to the wound, to preserve important collaterals, and, in advanced cases, to utilize collaterals for revascularization (Table 7.3).

Table 7.3 Important collateral pathways in peripheral artery disease.

Level of disease	Collateral pathway	Clinical significance
Aorto-iliac	IMA-IIA Lumbar-IIA Lumbar-Cx Iliac	Angiographic visualization Preserving collaterals in case of restenosis
Superficial femoral	PFA-popliteal	Angiographic visualization Preserving collaterals in case of restenosis
Popliteal 'trifurcation'	Geniculate arteries	Angiographic visualization
Tibioperoneal	ACA, PCA	Access for revascularization
Pedal	Plantar loop	Access for revascularization Angiosome concept

IMA, inferior mesenteric artery; IIA, internal iliac artery; Cx, circumflex; PFA, profunda femoral artery; ACA, anterior communicating artery; PCA, posterior communicating artery.

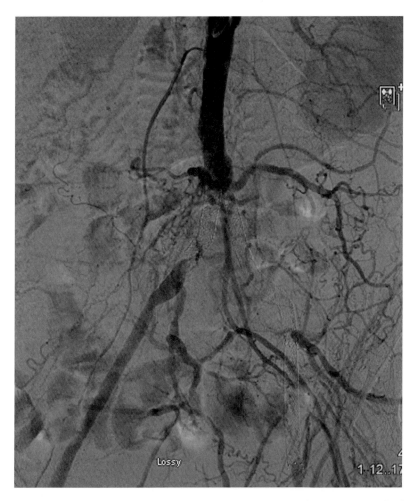

Figure 7.1 Aorto-iliac angiography in a patient with right common iliac artery and left common and external iliac artery occlusions. The inferior mesenteric artery and lumbar collaterals reconstitute vessels distal to the occlusions.

For *aorto-iliac occlusions*, the common femoral artery (CFA) is often reconstituted via pre-existing lumbar arteries to the circumflex iliac artery. Internal iliac arteries are usually reconstituted via the inferior mesenteric artery and lumbar collateral pathways [13]. Thus, angiography optimized to visualize the reconstituted segments requires placing the angiographic catheter cephalad to the inferior mesenteric artery and pertinent lumbar artery origins (Figure 7.1).

For *SFA occlusions*, the popliteal artery is reconstituted by the profunda femoral artery [13] (Figure 7.2). When antegrade access is obtained with the tip of the sheath in the SFA, the reconstituted popliteal artery may be difficult to

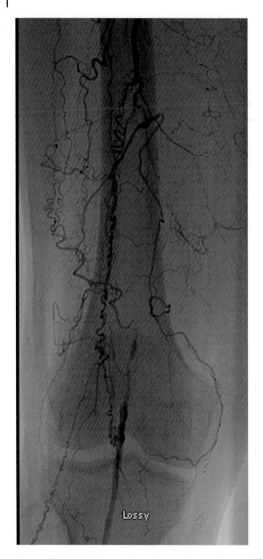

Figure 7.2 Right lower extremity angiogram in a patient with superficial femoral artery occlusion. The above-knee popliteal artery is reconstituted via collaterals from the profunda femoral artery.

visualize as contrast injections occur caudal to the donor collaterals. If the profunda is occluded, collaterals may come from the internal iliac or mesenteric arteries (Figure 7.3).

In the case of *popliteal occlusions extending into the origins of the tibioperoneal arteries*, geniculate collaterals typically reconstitute the tibioperoneal

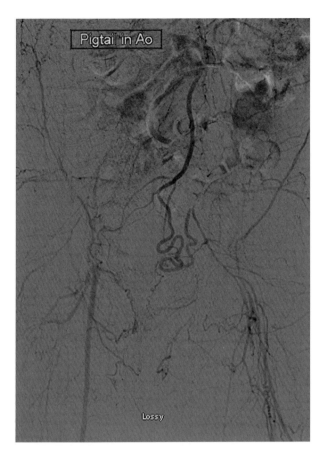

Figure 7.3 Aortography in a patient with an infrarenal aortic occlusion involving a prior aorto-bifemoral graft. The infrainguinal vessels are reconstituted via the superior mesenteric artery.

vessels [13]. Collateral pathways below the knee often require arteriogenesis, or generation of new arterial conduits, rather than utilization of pre-existing anastamotic pathways [14] (Figure 7.4). Two important, naturally occurring anastomoses below the knee include the anterior communicating artery (connects the anterior tibial and peroneal arteries above the ankle) and the posterior communicating artery (connects the posterior tibial and peroneal arteries above the ankle) [13] (Figure 7.5).

The anatomy of vascular angiosomes of the foot and the plantar arch are important concepts for the endovascular interventionalist (Figure 7.6). The posterior tibial artery gives rise to lateral plantar artery, which has an anastomosis with the dorsalis pedis artery to form the plantar arch (Figure 7.7) [13]. Variations of the plantar arch include an incomplete arch with varying degrees

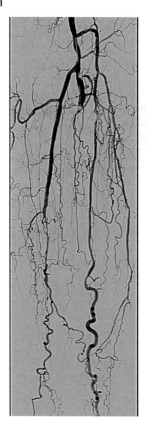

Figure 7.4 Left below-knee angiography in a patient with occlusions of the posterior tibial, anterior tibial, and peroneal arteries. Unnamed collaterals formed via arteriogenesis to supply conduits for pedal perfusion.

of contribution from the dorsalis pedis and lateral plantar artery. Additionally, the peroneal artery may rise to the dorsalis pedis through the lateral perforating branch [13] (Figure 7.8). The heel may be supplied via either the posterior tibial or peroneal artery [15]. Establishing direct flow into the angiosome of a wound may improve healing in patients with CLI [16, 17].

Technical Background

Preprocedural Imaging

After the decision has been made to pursue revascularization for claudication, diagnostic testing can identify the level and extent of PAD. Such information provides insight into risk–benefit assessment, projected long-term patency, and planning for the endovascular procedure. In addition to the history and

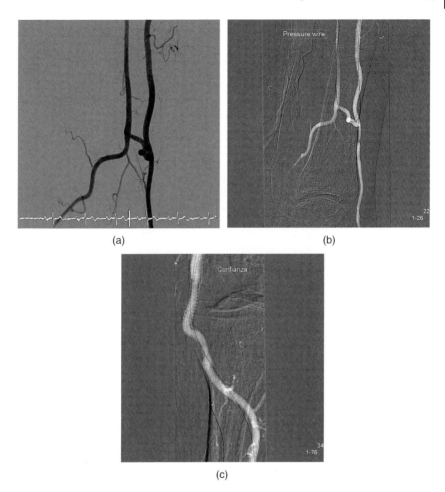

Figure 7.5 (a) Selective left anterior tibial angiogram showing anterior communicating artery reconstituting an occluded peroneal artery. (b) A guidewire and microcatheter have traversed the anterior tibial artery and anterior communicating artery to access the peroneal artery retrograde. (c) Interventional wire at proximal cap of peroneal occlusion.

physical examination, physiologic studies provide information on the level of disease as well as establishing a pre-procedural baseline, which is useful for post-procedural surveillance. Duplex ultrasonography can be useful in assessing suitability of the CFA for access and in defining the extent of SFA disease. Computed tomography (CT) and magnetic resonance (MR) angiography visualize pelvic vessels well and can refine pre-procedural anatomic definition of the femoral arteries [18]. Tibioperoneal arteries are more challenging to assess, even with the highest quality duplex ultrasound. CT angiography, MR

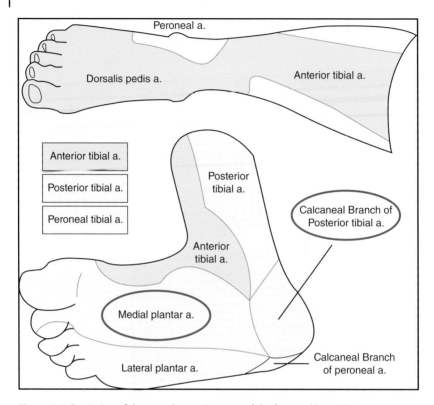

Figure 7.6 Depiction of the vascular angiosomes of the foot and lower leg.

angiography, catheter-based angiography, physical examination, and distal hemodyamic assessments (toe pressure, toe plethysmography, transmetatarsal and ankle pulse volume recordings, and ankle pressures) may have more clinical utility.

Access

The most appropriate access site for endovascular interventions is influenced by the target lesion location, quality of the access vessel, anticipated needs for crossing and treating (support and arteriotomy size) the involved segments, and the length of the equipment available (wires, catheters, balloons, and stents) (Table 7.4). In general, the ipsilateral retrograde femoral approach is ideal for common iliac and proximal to mid-external iliac lesions. The contralateral retrograde femoral approach is preferred for lesions in the contralateral internal iliac, distal external iliac, CFA, profunda, SFA, popliteal, and sometimes infrapopliteal arteries [19]. Additional options for the mid-distal SFA, popliteal, and infrapopliteal arteries are ipsilateral antegrade CFA access

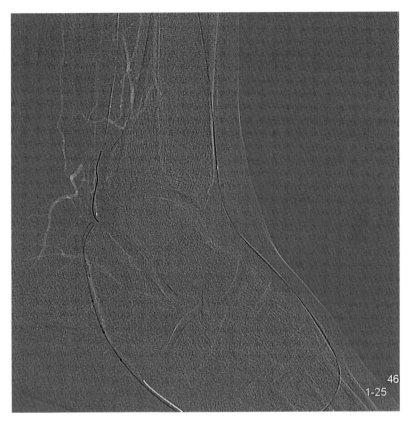

Figure 7.7 Demonstration of the plantar arch. An interventional guidewire and microcatheter have traversed the anterior tibial artery and dorsalis pedis artery into the lateral plantar artery (plantar arch) to facilitate true lumen re-entry of the wire in the distal posterior tibial artery.

and retrograde pedal access via the dorsalis pedis or posterior tibial arteries. The latter two approaches are often chosen in cases where difficulty in crossing tibioperoneal occlusions is anticipated (Figure 7.9).

Anticoagulation

For both coronary and peripheral interventions, unfractionated heparin (UFH) has been the traditional anticoagulant of choice. Although the effect of a given dose in an individual patient is largely unpredictable due to variable bioavailability, the level of anticoagulation is easily monitored via the activated clotting time (ACT). A study in 2010 showed that during peripheral vascular interventions, a higher total heparin dose ($\geq$60 U/kg) and a peak procedural ACT $\geq$ 250 seconds were predictors of post-procedural bleeding events. Moreover, the

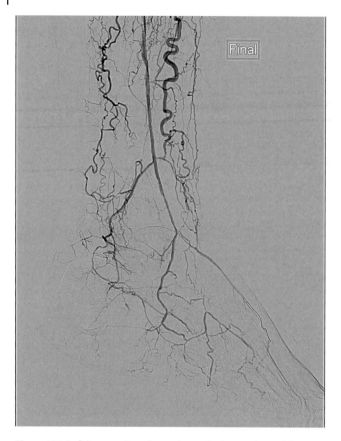

Figure 7.8 Left lower extremity angiography in a patient with congenital anomaly of peroneal artery supplying the dorsalis pedis artery. Note the interventional wire in the dorsalis pedis artery following successful peroneal reconstruction.

technical and procedural success in patients who received a total heparin dose < 60 U/kg ($n = 2161$) and ≥ 60 U/kg ($n = 2582$) was high, and the rate of thromboembolic complications was low with no difference between groups. These findings suggest that use of weight-based heparin dosing (initially, up to 60 U/kg) with a target ACT of 200–250 seconds may result in good procedural outcomes with decreased bleeding rates in peripheral vascular interventions as compared with higher ACT goals [20].

Potential alternatives to UFH include low-molecular-weight heparins and the direct thrombin inhibitor bivalirudin. From a cost perspective, UFH is far less expensive than its alternatives. It additionally has the unique benefit of complete reversibility with protamine sulfate, an important consideration in cases where there may be increased risk of catastrophic bleeding,

Table 7.4 Recommended arterial access sites, depending on lesion location.

Lesion location	Preferred access site	Alternative access sites
Aortic bifurcation	Bilateral retrograde CFA	Bilateral brachial or radial arteries
Common iliac artery	Ipsilateral retrograde CFA	Contralateral retrograde CFA, brachial, radial
Proximal and mid-external iliac artery	Ipsilateral retrograde CFA	Contralateral retrograde CFA, brachial, or radial
Distal external iliac artery	Contralateral retrograde CFA	Brachial or radial
CFA	Contralateral retrograde CFA	Brachial, radial, or popliteal
Proximal SFA	Contralateral retrograde CFA	Ipsilateral antegrade CFA, brachial, popliteal, retrograde pedal
Mid or distal SFA	Contralateral retrograde CFA	Ipsilateral antegrade CFA, brachial, or popliteal
Profunda femoris artery	Contralateral retrograde CFA	Brachial
Popliteal artery	Contralateral retrograde CFA	Ipsilateral antegrade CFA or ipsilateral retrograde pedal
Infrapopliteal	Ipsilateral antegrade	Contralateral CFA or retrograde pedal

CFA, common femoral artery; SFA, superficial femoral artery.

potentially from non-compressible sites. The advantages of direct thrombin inhibitors over UFH include a more specific and potent inhibition of thrombin [19]. The direct thrombin inhibitor bivalrudin was tested in the APPROVE trial and shown to be safe and efficacious in a variety of peripheral interventions [21]. Platelet glycoprotein IIb/IIIa receptor inhibitors have not been tested in aorto-iliac interventions and cannot be currently recommended. However, these agents as well as localized low-dose thrombolytics may be useful as bailout strategies in case of peri-procedural thromboembolic complications [22].

Antiplatelet Management

All patients undergoing peripheral revascularization should be on an antiplatelet agent. If aspirin is not tolerated, clopidogrel may be used as an alternative. In patients undergoing percutaneous transluminal angioplasty (PTA) not on antiplatelet drugs, 325 mg of oral aspirin (or 300–600 mg of clopidogrel in case of aspirin intolerance) may be given prior to gaining femoral access. There is no consensus regarding the use of pre-procedural clopidogrel loading for

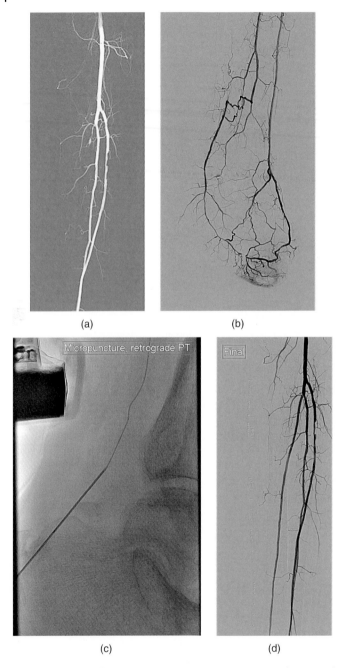

(a)

(b)

Micropuncture, retrograde PT

Final

(c)

(d)

Figure 7.9 (a, b) Left below-knee angiogram in a patient with a wound on the lateral foot following transmetatarsal amputation. (c) Access needle and wire in the left posterior tibial artery. (d) Final angiogram following posterior tibial artery reconstruction.

patients undergoing PTA who are on chronic aspirin treatment. Pre-procedure dual antiplatelet therapy, if not mandatory for a coronary indication, should be avoided in patients undergoing recanalization of an iliac total occlusion, because it might jeopardize surgical bailout of complications such as a perforation. Following successful iliac stenting, in addition to lifelong aspirin, clopidogrel is frequently administered with a loading dose of 300–600 mg, followed by a maintenance dose of 75 mg/day for at least 1 month [23]. The Clopidogrel and Aspirin in the Management of Peripheral Endovascular Revascularization (CAMPER) study was designed to test the utility of dual antiplatelet therapy compared with a single antiplatelet agent alone in patients undergoing endovascular lower extremity intervention. Unfortunately, poor enrollment in the CAMPER trial ultimately led to early study termination by the sponsor [24]. Therefore, the optimal post-procedure antithrombotic regimen remains uncertain. The pilot ePAD trial may add to our knowledge base in this arena (clinicaltrials.gov #NCT01802775).

Radiation

Ionizing radiation makes peripheral interventions possible but poses a significant health risk to the patient and operator. The effects of radiation are dose-dependent and may be minimized by limiting exposure, proper patient positioning, equipment calibration, and appropriate shielding. In a retrospective study, 382 peripheral interventions were analyzed and it was found that the dose area product (DAP) was significantly higher for procedures performed in the pelvis than in thigh procedures (179.6 vs. 63.2 Gy cm^2; $P < 0.0001$) and below-knee procedures (179.6 vs. 28.9 Gy cm^2; $P < 0.0001$), despite shorter fluoroscopy times (11.8 vs. 16.4 minutes; $P < 0.0001$ and 11.1 vs. 31.06 minutes; $P < 0.0001$, respectively) owing to greater tissue penetration in the pelvis. Procedure access site affected radiation dose as well with contralateral retrograde CFA access, resulting in a higher DAP than antegrade CFA access (112.2 vs 42.6 Gy cm^2; $P < 0.0001$). In a multivariable analysis, anatomic location of the procedure showed the strongest association with radiation dose ($P < 0.0001$), with aorto-iliac interventions associated with significantly higher doses than infrainguinal procedures [25].

Chronic Total Occlusions

In the case of chronic total occlusions, crossing the lesion in the sub-intimal space is a frequent scenario at any vascular segment. Various techniques and approaches have been described, all of which have advantages or disadvantages to achieve this goal. To facilitate re-entry of the guidewire into the true lumen, specific re-entry devices have been introduced (Table 7.5) [26]. In addition to dedicated re-entry devices, joining antegrade and retrograde sub-intimal spaces to allow access to the true lumen is an alternative technique (Figure 7.10) [27].

Table 7.5 Re-entry devices for endovascular intervention.

Device	Company
Outback	Cordis
Pioneer	Volcano
Viance	Ev3
OffRoad	Boston Scientific

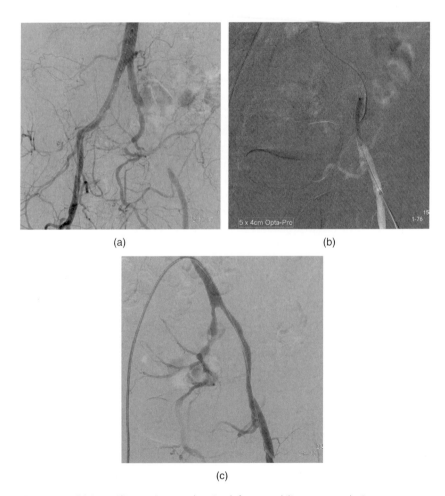

(a)

(b)

(c)

Figure 7.10 (a) Aorto-iliac angiogram showing left external iliac artery occlusion. (b) Retrograde balloon inflation to facilitate the antegrade wire entry into the true lumen distal to the occlusion. (c) Final angiography following left external iliac artery revascularization.

Clinical Evidence for Peripheral Intervention

Aorto-Iliac Interventions

The assessment of clinically significant stenoses is often based on combining information from history, physical examination, and non-invasive imaging. If diagnostic uncertainty remains, measuring a translesional pressure gradient has a class 1, level of evidence B recommendation [12]. In 2007, The TransAtlantic Inter-Society Consensus Working Group II (TASC II) formulated recommendations for revascularization of aorto-iliac lesions based on anatomic complexity. For simple lesions (TASC II A/B) the endovascular treatment was recommended as therapy of choice, whereas for complex stenoses/occlusions (TASC II C/D lesions), surgery was preferred (Table 7.6) [22].

Over the ensuing several years, endovascular interventional technologies and operator experience advanced dramatically, leading many to question the utility of the original TASC II recommendations, particularly for TASC C and D lesions [28]. In light of this controversy, the Society for Cardiovascular Angiography and Interventions has recently proposed expert consensus guidelines for endovascular aorto-iliac interventions [29]. These recommendations state that type C lesions offer satisfactory results with endovascular methods, such that this approach is preferred first, unless an open revascularization is

Table 7.6 TransAtlantic Inter-Society Consensus (TASC II) morphologic stratification of iliac lesions.

Lesion type	Description
A	Single stenosis of CIA or EIA < 3 cm long (unilateral or bilateral)
B	Single stenosis 3–10 cm long, not extending into CFA Two stenoses of CIA or EIA < 5 cm long, not involving CFA
	Unilateral CIA occlusion
C	Bilateral stenosis of CIA and/or EIA 5–10 cm long, not involving CFA
	Unilateral EIA occlusion not involving CFA
	Unilateral EIA stenosis extending into CFA
	Bilateral CIA occlusion
D	Diffuse stenosis of the entire CIA, EIA, and CFA > 10 cm long
	Unilateral occlusion of CIA and EIA
	Bilateral EIA occlusion
	Iliac stenosis adjacent to aortic or iliac aneurysm

CIA, common iliac artery; EIA, external iliac artery; CFA, common femoral artery.

required for other associated lesions in the same anatomic area. For type D lesions, surgical bypass is still the preferred treatment modality for revascularization. However, with improved operator techniques and newer re-entry devices, experienced endovascular specialists are able to approach TASC D lesions percutaneously. The impetus to pursue endovascular treatment for even complex aorto-iliac disease is strengthened by the risks of aortofemoral bypass, which carries a perioperative mortality approaching 4% [30] and the reasonable patency of percutaneous revascularization in this segment, as discussed below. In the end, treatment decisions need to be based on a comprehensive evaluation of the individual patient and characteristics of the target vessel and target lesion.

Angioplasty vs. Stent

A randomized trial of 279 patients with claudication compared primary stenting (stenting regardless of initial angioplasty result) with angioplasty and provisional stenting (stenting for suboptimal angioplasty result) [31]. Over a mean follow-up of 9.3 months, improvements in claudication and patency approached 80% and were similar between the two groups [31]. In the provisional stenting arm, stenting was performed in 43% of patients. These results suggest that provisional stenting is an acceptable strategy, but that stenting will be increasingly necessary as anatomic complexity increases.

Overall, observational data suggest favorable outcomes for aorto-iliac stenting for symptomatic PAD. In one observational study of 365 patients in whom 505 iliac lesions were treated with stents, primary patency at 8 years was 74% [32]. A separate study reported a re-intervention rate of 18% at 5.6 years of follow-up in patients undergoing iliac stenting [33]. Complications occur in up to 4% of cases and include vascular access complications, iliac perforation, and distal embolization [34]. These studies underscore the long-term durability of iliac stenting, which approaches that achieved with aortobifemoral bypass surgery, where 5- and 10-year patency rates of 80–90% are reported [35].

In deciding between self-expanding nitinol stents and balloon-expandable stents, there is no head-to-head comparative evidence. For aorto-iliac bifurcation lesions, balloon-expandable stents (covered or uncovered) are often placed bilaterally in the common iliac arteries (CIAs) extending slightly into the distal abdominal aorta (using a stent with diameter matched to iliac vessel diameter) for precise reconstruction of the bifurcation. Distal external iliac artery (EIA) lesions may be best treated with self-expanding stents because there is greater movement at this site owing to its proximity to the hip joint (using a stent with diameter 1–2 mm larger than vessel diameter). Significant size mismatch between the proximal and distal reference vessel segments also favors the use of a self-expanding stent (sizing stent to proximal reference vessel diameter)

[22]. However, in many cases of iliac revascularization, operator preference is the major determining factor in stent choice.

Polytetrafluoroethylene (PTFE)-Covered Versus Bare Metal Balloon-Expandable Stents

In the past, covered stents had been reserved for iliac aneurysms, arteriovenous fistulae, and iatrogenic perforations. Recent studies have provided encouraging results comparing PTFE-covered stents with balloon-expandable bare metal stents for aorto-iliac lesions. The COBEST (a Comparison of Covered versus Bare Expandable stents for the Treatment of Aorto-iliac Occlusive Disease) trial randomized 168 iliac arteries (TASC B–D) to balloon-expandable, PTFE (ePTFE)-covered stents or an array of balloon-expandable bare metal stents [36]. The primary outcome was binary restenosis > 50% at 18 months. Restenosis occurred in eight out of 82 limbs in the covered stent group and 20 out of 86 limbs in the bare metal stent group. There was a statistically significant advantage in freedom from restenosis in the covered stent group (hazard ratio [HR] = 0.35; 95% confidence interval (CI): 0.15–0.82; P = 0.02). This benefit was seen primarily in TASC C/D lesions (HR = 0.136; 95% CI: 0.042–0.442). There was no significant difference across groups for the less complex TASC B lesions (HR = 0.748; 95% CI: 0.235–2.386) [37]. A limitation of this study was the inclusion of seven types of stent platforms in the non-covered bare metal stent arm.

A disadvantage of ePTFE-covered stents is the requirement for relatively larger sheath sizes for their delivery. Another disadvantage of covered stents is that treatment of certain lesions may require coverage of major side branches, including the internal iliac artery and/or major collaterals. With non-covered stents, the majority of these side branches will maintain patency, and in cases where patency is lost, endovascular rescue is often possible.

The ACCF/AHA guidelines and the TASC II guidelines recommend primary stenting in CIAs and EIAs as class IB and class IC indications, respectively. With respect to CFA interventions, stenting should be avoided whenever possible, in order to prevent crushing, high rates of stent fracture, and to preserve future vascular access [38].

Femoropopliteal Interventions

The previously mentioned, TASC II guidelines also classified femoropopliteal lesions and corresponding recommended therapies (Table 7.7). Since the publication of the TASC II document, endovascular techniques and operator experience have advanced such that procedural success can be achieved in the vast majority of complex lesions, including TASC C/D lesions. However, the challenge is long-term patency at this anatomic level. The Society for

Table 7.7 TransAtlantic Inter-Society Consensus Working Group II (TASC II) classification for femoropopliteal peripheral artery disease.

Classification	Lesion(s)	Recommendation
Type A lesions	Single stenosis ≤ 10 cm in length	Endovascular therapy is the treatment of choice for TASC A lesions
	Single occlusion ≤ 5 cm in length	
Type B lesions	Multiple lesions (stenoses or occlusions), each ≤ 5 cm	Endovascular therapy is the preferred treatment for type B lesions; the patient's comorbidities, fully informed patient preference, and the local operator's long-term success rates must be considered when making treatment recommendations for type B and type C lesions
	Single stenosis or occlusion ≤ 15 cm not involving the infrageniculate popliteal artery	
	Single or multiple lesions in the absence of continuous tibial vessels to improve inflow for a distal bypass	
	Heavily calcified occlusion ≤ 5 cm in length	
	Single popliteal stenosis	
Type C lesions	Multiple stenoses or occlusions totaling ≥ 5 cm with or without heavy calcification	Surgery is the preferred treatment for good-risk patients with type C lesions; the patient's comorbidities, fully informed patient preference, and the local operator's long-term success rates must be considered when making treatment recommendations for type B and type C lesions
	Recurrent stenoses or occlusions that need treatment after two endovascular interventions	
Type D lesions	Chronic total occlusions of the CFA or SFA > 20 cm involving the popliteal artery	Surgery is the treatment of choice for TASC D lesions
	Chronic total occlusion of the popliteal artery and proximal trifurcation vessels	

Source: Adapted from Norgren *et al.* [38].
CFA, common femoral artery; SFA, superficial femoral artery.

Cardiovascular Angiography and Interventions has more recently formulated appropriateness criteria for endovascular femoropopliteal interventions [29].

Angioplasty versus Stenting

The femoropopliteal segment is an extremely challenging area with respect to restenosis and re-occlusion after endovascular treatment. During ambulation, various forces are exerted on this vessel, including flexion, longitudinal and lateral compression, and torsion, which may influence long-term outcomes after endovascular treatment. Restenosis rates after PTA vary between 40% and 60% at 1 year, with up to 70% failure at 1 year after angioplasty of lesions > 10 cm [39]. Balloon-expanding endovascular stents in the femoropopliteal segment resolved the problems of early elastic recoil, residual stenosis, and flow-limiting dissections after plain balloon angioplasty, but several randomized controlled trials failed to demonstrate a beneficial effect of SFA stenting with stainless steel stents compared with plain balloon angioplasty [40–43]. Self-expanding nitinol stents have been compared with angioplasty alone in the femoropopliteal segments in randomized trials [34]. In summary, short lesions with a mean length of up to 6 cm seem to respond well to PTA. Lesions of a mean of > 8 cm showed better patency rates after nitinol stent implantation. In addition to improvement in patency, a benefit in patients-oriented outcomes for nitinol stenting over angioplasty alone has been suggested. For example, in a randomized trial of 104 patients with claudication or CLI, treadmill-walking distance was significantly better in the group randomized to stenting [44].

Drug-Eluting Stents in Femoropopliteal Arteries

Suboptimal patency of endovascular treatment of the femoropopliteal arteries created interest in drug-coated stent (DCS) technology with the hopes of improved patency. Only a few studies have been conducted on the use of DCS in the femoropopliteal arteries.

Sirolimus-Coated Cordis Self-Expandable Stent (SIROCCO) II was a multicenter, double-blind study of a sirolimus-eluting self-expanding nitinol stent compared with the same platform bare-metal stent (BMS) in the SFA. The mean lesion length in the 93 patients included was 8.3 cm. At 24 months, the in-stent restenosis rate by duplex ultrasound in the DCS group was 22.9% versus 21.1% in the BMS group (P = NS). The lack of a statistically significant difference between the two groups may be related to the unexpectedly low restenosis rate in the BMS group [45].

The Safety and Efficacy Study of the Dynalink-E Everolimus Eluting Peripheral Stent System (STRIDES) was a prospective, non-randomized, single-arm trial using an everolimus-eluting self-expanding nitinol stent in 104 patients with femoropopliteal disease and a mean lesion length of 9.0 cm [46]. Primary patency rates were 94% and 68% at 6 and 12 months, respectively, and plain radiographic examination of 122 stents revealed no evidence of stent fracture after 12 months. However, a retrospective comparison with the Vienna Absolute trial demonstrated nearly identical restenosis rates with the corresponding BMS [44].

In 2011, the 12-month results of the Zilver PTX Randomized Study were reported [47]. This prospective, randomized, multicenter trial with 479 patients (Zilver PTX, n = 241; angioplasty, n = 238) had two randomization protocols. First, the patients were randomized to treatment with either traditional PTA or the paclitaxel-coated Zilver stent. In the angioplasty group, about 120 (50%) patients had suboptimal angioplasty and underwent secondary randomization to provisional stenting with a Zilver PTX (n – 61) or bare metal Zilver (n = 59). Mean lesion lengths were 63 and 66 mm, respectively. The primary patency rates at 12 months were 83.1% in the Zilver PTX group and 65.3% in the optimal PTA group ($P < 0.001$). To examine the drug effect, the investigators conducted a head-to-head comparison of secondary randomization to provisional stenting with Zilver PTX or BMS and found 12-month patency rates of 89.9% and 73%, respectively ($P=0.01$). Stent fractures were rare in both Zilver PTX and BMS patients, with an overall rate of 0.9% through 12 months, and no fractures resulted in clinical sequelae [47]. The 24-month update of this randomized trial reported that the primary patency remained significantly improved in the Zilver PTX arm compared with patients with successful PTA (74.8% vs. 26.5%; $P < 0.01$) [48].

Drug-Coated Balloon (DCB) Therapy in Femoropopliteal Disease

There have been several completed randomized studies comparing DCB with standard balloons that used angiographic surrogate end-points, the THUNDER (Taxan With Short Time for Contact for Reduction of Restenosis in Distal Arteries) trial and the Femoral Paclitaxel trial [49, 50]. In THUNDER, 154 patients with femoropopliteal disease were randomized to standard balloon angioplasty, standard balloons with paclitaxel in the contrast medium, or paclitaxel-coated balloons. There was a statistically significant difference favoring the paclitaxel-coated balloon arm in the primary outcome of 6-month late lumen loss [49]. Another randomized trial of 87 patients showed similar improvements in 6-month late lumen loss for paclitaxel balloon therapy versus standard angioplasty in straightforward femoropopliteal disease [50].

Early results from a larger trial, LEVANT 2, have been presented. The study was designed to look at 12-month outcomes in 476 patients with stenotic femoropopliteal arteries randomized 2:1 to either a drug-eluting balloon or standard balloon angioplasty. At 6 months, freedom from restenosis was significantly more common in the DCB group, and rates of target lesion revascularization (TLR) were identical in the two groups. Binary restenosis, a secondary end-point, was halved in the DCB group compared with the standard angioplasty group (17% vs. 34%, $P < 0.001$) [51].

Ongoing studies include in.PACT SFA (Randomized Trial of IN.PACT [Paclitaxel] Admiral DEB vs Standard PTA for the Treatment of Atherosclerotic Lesions in the SFA and/or Proximal Popliteal Artery) and the ILLUMENATE trial (a multicenter, prospective, randomized trial evaluating the safety and effectiveness of the Stellarex drug-coated angioplasty balloon vs. an uncoated standard angioplasty balloon in the treatment of *de novo* or restenotic lesions in the superficial femoral or popliteal artery).

Covered Stents in Femoropopliteal Disease

Data on the use of covered, self-expanding stents in the femoropopliteal territory are limited and primarily involve several iterations of Viabahn stents (WL Gore & Associates, Flagstaff, AZ, USA). In a small randomized study, use of a PTFE-covered Viabahn stent had similar 12- and 24-month patency compared with surgical femoral-to-above knee bypass [52]. At the 4-year follow-up, there was no difference between the two treatment strategies with regard to primary or secondary patency [53]. The VIBRANT (Viabahn Versus Bare Nitinol Stent in the Treatment of Long Lesion [≥8 cm] Superficial Femoral Artery Occlusive Disease) trial compared treatment with Viabahn and bare metal nitinol stents. There was no difference in outcome between the two treatment groups, with poor 12-month primary patency for both the Viabahn and bare nitinol stents (53% vs. 58%; P = NS) [54].

Newer generation Viabahn stents have also been investigated. A single-arm, multicenter prospective registry, VIPER (Viabahn Endoprosthesis with Heparin Bioactive Surface in the Treatment of Superficial Femoral Artery Obstructive Disease), evaluated the heparin-bonded Viabahn in 120 patients with long SFA stenosis or occlusion (mean lesion length = 19 cm) [55]. The 12-month primary patency in VIPER was 73%, suggesting a potentially favorable impact of the heparin bioactive surface on stent patency. Most recently, the VIASTAR (Viabahn Endoprosthesis with PROPATEN Bioactive Surface [VIA] versus Bare Nitinol Stent in the Treatment of Long Lesions in Superficial Femoral Artery Occlusive Disease) trial compared the heparin-bonded Viabahn-covered stent with a BMS for the treatment of complex femoropopliteal lesions. A total of 141 patients with symptomatic peripheral artery disease were assigned to treatment with a Viabahn-covered stent or BMS. In the per-protocol analysis, the 12-month primary patency rate was 78.1% in the Viabahn group versus 53.5% in the BMS group. For lesions ≥ 20 cm, the apparent benefit was even greater, with a primary patency rate of 73.3% for Viabahn versus 33.3% for BMS [56]. Such a patency rate for long lesions is encouraging. However, the most concerning complication of covered stent use in the femoropopliteal arteries is the potential for stent thrombosis that can present as acute limb ischemia. While the recent results with the latest Viabahn stent are promising, all the

Table 7.8 Available atherectomy devices for peripheral arterial interventions.

Device	Company	Mechanism
Silverhawk	Ev3	Excisional atherectomy
Diamondback	Cardiovascular Systems Inc.	Orbital atherectomy
Excimer Laser	Spectranetics	Laser ablation
Jetstream Pathway	Medrad	Rotational atherectomy with aspiration

studies were underpowered and too limited in duration of follow-up to assess for this catastrophic outcome.

Atherectomy

The theoretical benefits of atherectomy are based on plaque removal or modification to facilitate successful revascularization. Currently, four main atherectomy systems are available: excisional atherectomy, orbital atherectomy, rotational atherectomy, and laser atherectomy (Table 7.8). Atherectomy is used in a variety of clinical situations based on operator preference. These include, but are not limited to, debulking or modifying heavily calcified lesions to allow for complete stent expansion, and primary treatment of obstructive disease at joints (CFA and popliteal artery) where stents might be more prone to fracture and adverse clinical sequelae.

Randomized data for peripheral atherectomy are sparse. Excisional atherectomy was studied in a small, randomized trial comparing 29 patients treated by filter-protected atherectomy with 29 patients treated with balloon angioplasty alone. Target lesion revascularization at 12 months was 16.7% versus 11.1%, respectively (P = NS). Secondary stenting was performed in 62% of the patients in the balloon angioplasty group versus 28% in the atherectomy group (P = 0.017). Thus, atherectomy offered no obvious improvement in clinical results compared with balloon angioplasty, apart from the reduced need for stents in this small, underpowered trial [57].

Observational evidence for orbital atherectomy in the femoropopliteal segments have suggested a reduced need for stents as well [58], and a randomized trial has shown similar results. In COMPLIANCE 360, 50 patients with symptomatic, calcific femoropopliteal disease were randomized to either orbital atherectomy with angioplasty or angioplasty alone [59]. Procedural success defined as < 30% residual stenosis was 87% in the atherectomy arm and 19% in the angioplasty arm (P < 0.001) [59]. Fewer stents were required in the atherectomy group (5.3%) than in the angioplasty-alone group (78%) [59]. There was not a statistically significant difference in restenosis at 12 months [59]. It is difficult to draw firm conclusions from this small trial; however, orbital atherectomy may have a role in achieving procedural success in calcified lesions.

Laser atherectomy was introduced over two decades ago for peripheral interventions. In a randomized comparison of excimer laser angioplasty versus angioplasty for the treatment of long SFA occlusions, excimer laser angioplasty was associated with decreased use of bailout stenting (42% vs. 59%) without improvement in 12-month patency [58]. Finally, rotational atherectomy with aspiration has been shown to be safe, although head-to-head comparisons with other devices are lacking. In a report of 172 prospectively enrolled patients with infrainguinal disease (31% total occlusions, mean lesion length = 2.7 cm), the procedural success was 99%, the 30-day major adverse event rate was 1%, and the 12-month restenosis rate was 38% [60].

Specialty Balloons

Cryoplasty, scoring, and cutting balloons are available for peripheral artery interventions. In a Cochrane review of seven trials comparing cryoplasty with conventional angioplasty in 478 patients with peripheral artery disease, cryoplasty was found to be safe but without a clear benefit in patency over a range of follow-up periods (3 months to 3 years) [61]. Data from scoring balloon angioplasty of femoropopliteal disease are limited at this time. The size matrix for cutting balloon angioplasty only supports treatment of very short lesions.

Tibioperoneal and Pedal Interventions

Tibioperoneal and pedal interventions are usually reserved for patients with Rutherford category 4, 5, and 6 CLI. Arterial access usually includes antegrade common femoral access but can also involve retrograde tibial access for recanalization of tibioperoneal occlusions. The use of collaterals and the plantar loop can also provide retrograde access for revascularization (Figure 7.7). More recently, skilled and experienced operators are even accessing transmetatarsal arteries [62]. Higher-intensity anticoagulation as compared with iliofemoral revascularization is anecdotally recommended to prevent thrombosis of the smaller below-knee vessels [63, 64].

Randomized trial data for tibioperoneal arteries is limited and is non-existent for endovascular pedal revascularization. There are no randomized trials comparing surgical with endovascular therapy at this anatomic level. Likewise, there are sparse randomized data comparing atherectomy with angioplasty alone, and no randomized trials comparing the various atherectomy devices with one another or with stenting. Randomized trials do exist for stenting versus angioplasty alone and for drug-eluting coronary stenting versus BMS and angioplasty alone. Given the lack of randomized data, decisions for below-knee revascularization rest largely on observational evidence, patient-specific factors, and operator experience.

In a meta-analysis of three randomized trials comparing drug-eluting stenting with either BMS or angioplasty alone, results were favorable for drug-eluting stenting [65]. This analysis included the trials YUKON-BTK (sirolimus-eluting stent vs. BMS), ACHILLES (sirolimus-eluting stent vs. angioplasty alone), and DESTINY (everolimus-eluting stent vs. BMS) [66–68]. In the pooled analysis of the 501 patients included in these trials, primary patency (80.0% vs 58.5%) and wound healing (76.8% vs. 59.7%) favored drug-eluting technology. Of note, mean lesion lengths were short (~15–30 mm among trials) and should be generalized with caution when treating longer occlusions commonly encountered below the knee.

In a meta-analysis comprising 18 observational studies and 640 patients who underwent stenting of a tibioperoneal artery for CLI, at 12 months, primary patency was observed in 78.9% (95% CI: 71.8–86%) and limb salvage in 96.4% (95% CI: 94.7–98.1%) [69]. Lesions and patient characteristics were not available in this analysis [69]. Due to the lack of randomization, comparison of stent types provides limited insight to guide therapeutic decisions [69].

Multiple atherectomy devices are available for treatment of tibioperoneal arteries, including laser ablation, excisional atherectomy, orbital atherectomy, and rotational atherectomy (Table 7.8). However, data with these technologies specific to below-knee intervention are sparse. Based on the available evidence, atherectomy of the tibioperoneal or pedal arteries is feasible and safe. For example, in a study of 52 below-knee arteries treated with excisional atherectomy, procedural success was 96%. Adjunctive angioplasty was performed in 29% of these lesions, and two required stent placement for flow-limiting dissection. The complication rate was 3% and consisted of target vessel occlusion. Six-month patency was 94.1 ± 3.3% [70].

The Laser Angioplasty for Critical Limb Ischemia phase 2 study enrolled 145 patients in whom infrapopliteal disease was treated with laser ablation. The procedural success was 86%, and the excellent 6-month limb salvage rate was 93% [71]. CALCIUM 360 was a randomized pilot study comparing orbital atherectomy followed by angioplasty with angioplasty alone in the treatment of 50 patients with CLI [72]. Of the lesions treated, 90.8% were tibioperoneal. There was no statistically significant difference in procedural success in the two arms in this underpowered pilot trial (93.1% for atherectomy/angioplasty vs. 82.4% for angioplasty alone; $P = 0.27$). However, a statistically significant benefit for orbital atherectomy was seen for freedom from target vessel revascularization at 1 year (93.3% vs. 68.4%, $P = 0.01$). There were no amputations in either group at 1 year.

Finally, many operators favor guiding revascularization decisions with the angiosome concept. That is, establishing in-line flow via arteries directly supplying a wound is thought to potentially improve wound healing as compared with the more traditional approach of restoring in-line flow below the knee of any vessel. In a retrospective observational study of 329 patients followed for a mean of 18 months, the 200 limbs in which percutaneous revascularization was achieved in the angiosome of interest had better outcomes than the 169 limbs for which revascularization was performed in a vessel not feeding the wound's angiosome [16]. After propensity score matching, freedom from amputation was 82% ± 5% for limbs that were successfully revascularized according to the angiosome concept but 68% ± 5% ($P = 0.01$) for the group with indirect revascularization [16].

Post-procedural Care

Aggressive cardiovascular risk factor reduction is a key component of post-procedural care to prevent cardiovascular events in patients with peripheral artery disease. Regular exercise should be an integral part of post-procedural care because of its well-established clinical benefit and because it provides a metric for detecting the progression of obstructive arterial disease. Supervised exercise therapy is an effective treatment for claudication and may offer additional benefits after lower extremity revascularization, although supervised exercise is not reimbursed [23].

In clinical practice, a frequently used pharmacotherapeutic strategy involves a 4-week course of dual antiplatelet therapy and subsequent indefinite therapy with aspirin [23]. However, unlike for coronary stenting, there is no evidence to guide antiplatelet management following lower extremity intervention. The duration and intensity of antiplatelet therapy must be balanced against the individual bleeding risk.

Surveillance strategies for patency depend on the patient's clinical indication for revascularization (CLI vs. claudication), the anatomic level that was treated, available assessment modalities (physical examination, physiologic studies, duplex ultrasonography, and cross-sectional imaging), and the expected consequence of restenosis. Guidelines from the ACCF/AHA recommend that patients with CLI who have been successfully treated be evaluated by a vascular specialist at least twice a year (class I, level of evidence C) [12]. These guidelines also state that patients with a history of CLI should receive instructions on self-surveillance (class I, level of evidence C) [12]. A class IIa, level of evidence C recommendation was given that patients with claudication or CLI who had undergone endovascular therapy could be evaluated in a surveillance program with physiologic assessment or imaging [12].

Conclusion

Endovascular therapy for PAD is rapidly progressing with technological advances and increased operator expertise, which allow for revascularization of increasingly complex anatomy with improvements in patency. Aorto-iliac intervention is particularly attractive as an alternative to aorto-femoral bypass due to lower morbidity and acceptable patency. Suboptimal durability plagues SFA revascularization, which should improve with emerging technology on the horizon. Percutaneous tibioperoneal and pedal revascularization is an important adjunctive therapy for limb salvage in patients with CLI. Due to lack of randomized trial data and the multitude of available devices for revascularization, decisions on how to perform endovascular intervention is currently based primarily on patient-specific factors and operator experience. Additional quality evidence in the field of endovascular therapy will better define this modality's role alongside medical therapy, supervised exercise, surgery, and wound care for patients with PAD.

References

1 Dotter CT, Judkins MP. Transluminal Treatment of Arteriosclerotic Obstruction. Description of a New Technic and a Preliminary Report of Its Application. Circulation. 1964; 30: 654–70.
2 Nowygrod R, Egorova N, Greco G, *et al.* Trends, complications, and mortality in peripheral vascular surgery. J Vasc Surg. 2006; 43(2): 205–16.
3 Rooke TW, Hirsch AT, Misra S, *et al.* 2011 ACCF/AHA Focused Update of the Guideline for the Management of Patients With Peripheral Artery Disease (updating the 2005 guideline): a report of the American College of Cardiology Foundation/American Heart Association Task Force on Practice Guidelines. J Am Coll Cardiol. 2011; 58(19): 2020–45.
4 Dormandy J, Heeck L, Vig S. The natural history of claudication: risk to life and limb. Semin Vasc Surg. 1999; 12(2): 123–37.
5 Murphy TP, Cutlip DE, Regensteiner JG, *et al.* Supervised exercise versus primary stenting for claudication resulting from aortoiliac peripheral artery disease: six-month outcomes from the claudication: exercise versus endoluminal revascularization (CLEVER) study. Circulation. 2012; 125(1): 130–9.
6 Belch J, Hiatt WR, Baumgartner I, *et al.* Effect of fibroblast growth factor NV1FGF on amputation and death: a randomised placebo-controlled trial of gene therapy in critical limb ischaemia. Lancet. 2011; 377(9781): 1929–37.
7 Becker F, Robert-Ebadi H, Ricco JB, *et al.* Chapter I: Definitions, epidemiology, clinical presentation and prognosis. Eur J Vasc Endovasc Surg. 2011; 42: S4–12.
8 Rueda CA, Nehler MR, *et al.* Patterns of artery disease in 450 patients undergoing revascularization for critical limb ischemia: implications for clinical trial design. J Vasc Surg. 2008; 47(5): 995–9 (discussion 9–1000).
9 Arain SA, White CJ. Endovascular therapy for critical limb ischemia. Vasc Med. 2008; 13(3): 267–79.

10 Romiti M, Albers M, Brochado-Neto, FC, *et al*. Meta-analysis of infrapopliteal angioplasty for chronic critical limb ischemia. J Vasc Surg. 2008; 47(5): 975–81.

11 Slovut DP, Sullivan TM. Critical limb ischemia: medical and surgical management. Vasc Med. 2008; 13(3): 281–91.

12 Anderson JL, Halperin JL, Albert NM, *et al*. Management of patients with peripheral artery disease (compilation of 2005 and 2011 ACCF/AHA guideline recommendations): a report of the American College of Cardiology Foundation/American Heart Association Task Force on Practice Guidelines. Circulation. 2013; 127(13): 1425–43.

13 Uflacker R. Atlas of Vascular Anatomy, 2nd edn. Philadelphia, PA: Lippencott, 2007.

14 Attanasio S, Snell J. Therapeutic angiogenesis in the management of critical limb ischemia: current concepts and review. Cardiol Rev. 2009; 17(3): 115–20.

15 Yan BP, Moran D, Hynes BG, *et al*. Advances in endovascular treatment of critical limb ischemia. Circulation journal : official journal of the Japanese Circ Soc. 2011; 75(4): 756–65.

16 Iida O, Soga Y, Hirano K, *et al*. Long-term results of direct and indirect endovascular revascularization based on the angiosome concept in patients with critical limb ischemia presenting with isolated below-the-knee lesions. J Vasc Surg. 2012; 55(2): 363–70 e5.

17 Neville RF, Attinger CE, Bulan EJ, Ducic I, Thomassen M, Sidawy AN. Revascularization of a specific angiosome for limb salvage: does the target artery matter? Ann Vasc Surg. 2009; 23(3): 367–73.

18 Lau JF, Weinberg MD, Olin JW. Peripheral artery disease. Part 1: clinical evaluation and noninvasive diagnosis. Nat Rev Cardiol. 2011; 8(7): 405–18.

19 Bhatt DL, ed. Guide to Peripheral and Cerebrovascular Intervention. London: Remedica, 2004.

20 Kasapis C, Gurm HS, Chetcuti SJ, *et al*. Defining the optimal degree of heparin anticoagulation for peripheral vascular interventions: insight from a large, regional, multicenter registry. Circ Cardiovasc Interv. 2010; 3(6): 593–601.

21 Allie DE, Hall P, Shammas NW, *et al*. The Angiomax Peripheral Procedure Registry of Vascular Events Trial (APPROVE): in-hospital and 30-day results. Jof Inv Cardiol. 2004; 16(11): 651–6.

22 Bonvini RF, Roffi M. Tools and techniques: Aorto-iliac and common femoral endovascular interventions. Eurointerventions. 2010; 6(2): 288–9.

23 Sobieszczyk P, Eisenhauer A. Management of patients after endovascular interventions for peripheral artery disease. Circulation. 2013; 128(7): 749–57.

24 Weinberg MD, Lau JF, Rosenfield K, Olin JW. Peripheral artery disease. Part 2: medical and endovascular treatment. Nat Rev Cardiol. 2011; 8(8): 429–41.

25 Segal E, Weinberg I, Leichter I, *et al*. Patient radiation exposure during percutaneous endovascular revascularization of the lower extremity. J Vasc Surg. 2013; 58(6): 1556–62.

26 Scheinert D, Schmidt A. Techniques for crossing iliac and aortoiliac CTOs. Endovasc Today. 2011: 39–43.

27 Rogers RK, Tsai T, Casserly IP. Novel application of the "CART" technique for endovascular treatment of external iliac artery occlusions. Catheter Cardio Inte. 2010; 75(5): 673–8.

28 Baril DT, Chaer RA, Rhee RY e#. Endovascular interventions for TASC II D femoropopliteal lesions. J Vasc Surg. 2010; 51(6): 1406–12.

29 Klein AJ, Feldman DN, Aronow HD *et al.* Appropriate use criteria: A society for cardiovascular angiography and interventions (SCAI) consensus statement for aorto-iliac arterial intervention. Catheter Cardiovasc Interv. 2014; 84(4): 520–8.

30 Clair D, Shah S, Weber J. Current state of diagnosis and management of critical limb ischemia. Curr Cardiol Rep. 2012; 14(2): 160–70.

31 Tetteroo E, van der Graaf Y, Bosch JL, *et al.* Randomised comparison of primary stent placement versus primary angioplasty followed by selective stent placement in patients with iliac-artery occlusive disease. Dutch Iliac Stent Trial Study Group. Lancet. 1998; 351(9110): 1153–9.

32 Murphy TP, Ariaratnam NS, Carney WI, Jr, *et al.* Aortoiliac insufficiency: long-term experience with stent placement for treatment. Radiology. 2004; 231(1): 243–9.

33 Klein WM, van der Graaf Y, Seegers J, *et al.* Long-term cardiovascular morbidity, mortality, and reintervention after endovascular treatment in patients with iliac artery disease: The Dutch Iliac Stent Trial Study. Radiology. 2004; 232(2): 491–8.

34 Schillinger M, Minar E. Percutaneous treatment of peripheral artery disease: novel techniques. Circulation. 2012; 126(20): 2433–40.

35 Hirsch AT, Haskal ZJ, Hertzer NR, *et al.* ACC/AHA Guidelines for the Management of Patients with Peripheral Arterial Disease (lower extremity, renal, mesenteric, and abdominal aortic): a collaborative report from the American Associations for Vascular Surgery/Society for Vascular Surgery, Society for Cardiovascular Angiography and Interventions, Society for Vascular Medicine and Biology, Society of Interventional Radiology, and the ACC/AHA Task Force on Practice Guidelines (writing committee to develop guidelines for the management of patients with peripheral arterial disease) – summary of recommendations. J Vasc Interv Radiol. 2006; 17(9): 1383–97 (quiz 98).

36 Mwipatayi BP, Thomas S, Wong J, *et al.* A comparison of covered vs bare expandable stents for the treatment of aortoiliac occlusive disease. J Vasc Surg. 2011; 54(6): 1561–70.

37 Grimme FA, Goverde PA, Van Oostayen JA, *et al.* Covered stents for aortoiliac reconstruction of chronic occlusive lesions. J Cardiovasc Surg. 2012; 53(3): 279–89.

38 Norgren L, Hiatt WR, Dormandy JA, *et al.* Inter-Society Consensus for the Management of Peripheral Arterial Disease (TASC II). J Vasc Surg. 2007; 45 Suppl S: S5–67.

39 Capek P, McLean GK, Berkowitz HD. Femoropopliteal angioplasty. Factors influencing long-term success. Circulation. 1991; 83(2 Suppl): I70–80.

40 Vroegindeweij D, Vos LD, Tielbeek AV, *et al.* Balloon angioplasty combined with primary stenting versus balloon angioplasty alone in femoropopliteal obstructions: A comparative randomized study. Cardiovasc Interv Radiol. 1997; 20(6): 420–5.

41 Grimm J, Muller-Hulsbeck S, Jahnke T, *et al.* Randomized study to compare PTA alone versus PTA with Palmaz stent placement for femoropopliteal lesions. J Vasc Interv Radiol. 2001; 12(8): 935–42.

42 Zdanowski Z, Albrechtsson U, Lundin A, *et al.* Percutaneous transluminal angioplasty with or without stenting for femoropopliteal occlusions? A randomized controlled study. Int Angiol. 1999; 18(4): 251–5.

43 Becquemin JP, Favre JP, Marzelle J, *et al.* Systematic versus selective stent placement after superficial femoral artery balloon angioplasty: a multicenter prospective randomized study. J Vasc Surg. 2003; 37(3): 487–94.

44 Schillinger M, Sabeti S, Loewe C, *et al.* Balloon angioplasty versus implantation of nitinol stents in the superficial femoral artery. N Engl J Med. 2006; 354(18): 1879–88.

45 Duda SH, Bosiers M, Lammer J, *et al.* Drug-eluting and bare nitinol stents for the treatment of atherosclerotic lesions in the superficial femoral artery: long-term results from the SIROCCO trial. J Endovasc Ther. 2006; 13(6): 701–10.

46 Lammer J, Bosiers M, Zeller T, *et al.* First clinical trial of nitinol self-expanding everolimus-eluting stent implantation for peripheral arterial occlusive disease. J Vasc Surg. 2011; 54(2): 394–401.

47 Dake MD, Ansel GM, Jaff MR, *et al.* Paclitaxel-eluting stents show superiority to balloon angioplasty and bare metal stents in femoropopliteal disease: twelve-month Zilver PTX randomized study results. Circ Cardiovasc Interv. 2011; 4(5): 495–504.

48 Dake MD, Ansel GM, Jaff MR, *et al.* Sustained safety and effectiveness of paclitaxel-eluting stents for femoropopliteal lesions: 2-year follow-up from the Zilver PTX randomized and single-arm clinical studies. J Am Coll Cardiol. 2013; 61(24): 2417–27.

49 Tepe G, Zeller T, Albrecht T, *et al.* Local delivery of paclitaxel to inhibit restenosis during angioplasty of the leg. N Engl J Med. 2008; 358(7): 689–99.

50 Werk M, Langner S, Reinkensmeier B, *et al.* Inhibition of restenosis in femoropopliteal arteries: paclitaxel-coated versus uncoated balloon: femoral paclitaxel randomized pilot trial. Circulation. 2008; 118(13): 1358–65.

51 Rosenfield K, ed. 6 Month Data of LEVANT 2 presented at TCT 2013. Transcatheter Cardiovascular Therapeutics 25th Annual Scientific Symposium; 2013 October 30, 2013; San Francisco, CA.

52 Kedora J, Hohmann S, Garrett W, *et al.* Randomized comparison of percutaneous Viabahn stent grafts vs prosthetic femoral-popliteal bypass in the treatment of superficial femoral arterial occlusive disease. J Vasc Surg. 2007; 45(1): 10–6; discussion 6.

53 McQuade K, Gable D, Pearl G, *et al.* Four-year randomized prospective comparison of percutaneous ePTFE/nitinol self-expanding stent graft versus prosthetic femoral-popliteal bypass in the treatment of superficial femoral artery occlusive disease. J Vasc Surg. 2010; 52(3): 584–90 (discussion 90–1, 91 e1-91 e7).

54 Geraghty PJ, Mewissen MW, Jaff MR, Ansel GM, VIBRANT Investigators. Three-year results of the VIBRANT trial of VIABAHN endoprosthesis versus bare nitinol stent implantation for complex superficial femoral artery occlusive disease. J Vasc Surg. 2013; 58(2): 386–95.

55 Saxon RR, Chervu A, Jones PA, *et al.* Heparin-bonded, expanded polytetrafluoroethylene-lined stent graft in the treatment of femoropopliteal artery disease: 1-year results of the VIPER (Viabahn Endoprosthesis with Heparin Bioactive Surface in the Treatment of Superficial Femoral Artery Obstructive Disease) trial. J Vasc Interv Radiol. 2013; 24(2): 165–73 (quiz 74).

56 Lammer J, Zeller T, Hausegger KA, *et al.* Heparin-bonded covered stents versus bare-metal stents for complex femoropopliteal artery lesions: the randomized VIASTAR trial (Viabahn endoprosthesis with PROPATEN bioactive surface [VIA] versus bare nitinol stent in the treatment of long lesions in superficial femoral artery occlusive disease). J Am Coll Cardiol. 2013; 62(15): 1320–7.

57 Shammas NW, Coiner D, Shammas GA, *et al.* Percutaneous lower-extremity arterial interventions with primary balloon angioplasty versus Silverhawk atherectomy and adjunctive balloon angioplasty: randomized trial. J Vasc Interv Radiol. 2011; 22(9): 1223–8.

58 Korabathina R, Mody KP, Yu J, *et al.* Orbital atherectomy for symptomatic lower extremity disease. Catheter Cardiovasc Interv. 2010; 76(3): 326–32.

59 Staniloae CS, Korabathina R. Orbital atherectomy: device evolution and clinical data. J Inv Cardiol. 2014; 26(5): 215–9.

60 Zeller T, Krankenberg H, Steinkamp H, *et al.* One-year outcome of percutaneous rotational atherectomy with aspiration in infrainguinal peripheral arterial occlusive disease: the multicenter pathway PVD trial. J Endovasc Ther. 2009; 16(6): 653–62.

61 McCaslin JE, Andras A, Stansby G. Cryoplasty for peripheral arterial disease. The Cochrane Database Syst Rev. 2013; 8: CD005507.

62 Manzi M, Palena LM. Retrograde percutaneous transmetatarsal artery access: new approach for extreme revascularization in challenging cases of critical limb ischemia. Cardiovasc Interv Radiol. 2013; 36(2): 554–7.

63 Lyden SP. Techniques and outcomes for endovascular treatment in the tibial arteries. J Vasc Surg. 2009; 50(5): 1219–23.

64 Falluji N, Mukherjee D. Contemporary management of infrapopliteal peripheral arterial disease. Angiology. 2011; 62(6): 490–9.

65 Katsanos K, Spiliopoulos S, Diamantopoulos A, *et al.* Systematic review of infrapopliteal drug-eluting stents: a meta-analysis of randomized controlled trials. Cardiovasc Interv Radiol. 2013; 36(3): 645–58.

66 Bosiers M, Scheinert D, Peeters P, *et al.* Randomized comparison of everolimus-eluting versus bare-metal stents in patients with critical limb ischemia and infrapopliteal arterial occlusive disease. J Vasc Surg. 2012; 55(2): 390–8.

67 Rastan A, Tepe G, Krankenberg H, *et al.* Sirolimus-eluting stents vs. bare-metal stents for treatment of focal lesions in infrapopliteal arteries: a double-blind, multi-centre, randomized clinical trial. Eur Heart J. 2011; 32(18): 2274–81.

68 Scheinert D, Katsanos K, Zeller T, *et al.* A prospective randomized multicenter comparison of balloon angioplasty and infrapopliteal stenting with the sirolimus-eluting stent in patients with ischemic peripheral arterial disease: 1-year results from the ACHILLES trial. J Am Coll Cardiol. 2012; 60(22): 2290–5.

69 Biondi-Zoccai GG, Sangiorgi G, Lotrionte M, *et al.* Infragenicular stent implantation for below-the-knee atherosclerotic disease: clinical evidence from an international collaborative meta-analysis on 640 patients. J Endovasc Ther. 2009; 16(3): 251–60.

70 Zeller T, Rastan A, Schwarzwalder U, *et al.* Midterm results after atherectomy-assisted angioplasty of below-knee arteries with use of the Silverhawk device. J Vasc Interv Radiol. 2004; 15(12): 1391–7.

71 Das TS. Excimer laser-assisted angioplasty for infrainguinal artery disease. J Endovasc Ther. 2009; 16(2 Suppl 2): II98–104.

72 Shammas NW, Lam R, Mustapha J, *et al.* Comparison of orbital atherectomy plus balloon angioplasty vs. balloon angioplasty alone in patients with critical limb ischemia: results of the CALCIUM 360 randomized pilot trial. J. Endovasc Ther. 2012; 19(4): 480–8.

8

Surgical Management of Peripheral Artery Disease
Julia Glaser[1] and Scott M. Damrauer[1, 2]

[1] Hospital of the University of Pennsylvania, Philadelphia, PA, USA
[2] Corporal Michael Crescent VA Medical Center, Philadelphia, PA, USA

When to Refer Patients with Claudication

Patients with peripheral artery disease (PAD) can present with a variety of complaints, including exertional leg symptoms, rest pain, foot ulcers, and gangrene (Table 8.1) [1]. Claudication, from the Latin *claudico* for limp, is thought of as the classic symptom of PAD, and has been defined as calf pain that begins while walking and is relieved by rest. Only a minority of patients with confirmed PAD, however, suffer from intermittent claudication. Rather, atypical leg symptoms predominate in most individuals [2].

Both the US Preventative Task Force and the Society for Vascular Surgery recommend against screening for PAD in the absence of symptoms [3]. Treatment of patients with incidentally discovered, but asymptomatic, PAD is aimed at reducing their overall risk of cardiovascular events, as PAD is a marker for advanced atherosclerotic disease. For patients with suspected PAD based on symptoms, however, referral to a vascular specialist for a thorough evaluation is warranted. There are numerous options for referral of these patients, including cardiologists, interventional radiologists, vascular medicine physicians, and vascular surgeons. These specialists can confirm the diagnosis, rule out rare disorders such as cystic adventitial disease or popliteal entrapment, and institute a comprehensive, individualized treatment plan for the patient.

As discussed in Chapter 6, medical management is the primary treatment for patients with claudication and comprises risk factor modification, supervised walking therapy, and secondary prevention of cardiovascular disease. These interventions are aimed at improving lower extremity symptoms, as well as reducing overall cardiovascular risk. The most important element of treatment of patients with claudication is to recognize that PAD is a marker of advanced

Peripheral Artery Disease, Second Edition. Edited by Emile R. Mohler and Michael R. Jaff.
© 2017 John Wiley & Sons Ltd. Published 2017 by John Wiley & Sons Ltd.

Table 8.1 Fontaine classification of vascular disease [1].

Stage	Description
I	Asymptomatic
II	Claudication
III	Ischemic rest pain
IV	Tissue loss (ischemic ulceration or necrosis)

atherosclerotic disease. These patients are at high risk for myocardial infarction and stroke, and absolutely merit secondary prevention regardless of whether their PAD is treated medically or with a procedure.

The goal of revascularization is to address symptoms, and, as such, revascularization for claudication is only appropriate for individuals with lifestyle-limiting or debilitating disease. This assessment is, by design, subjective and can vary from patient to patient. Consider a mail carrier whose claudication limits him to walking 100 yards at a time, severely limiting his ability to perform his job. Clearly, this patient would benefit from an improvement in his claudication, and he therefore merits revascularization. An older patient with chronic obstructive pulmonary disease who claudicates but whose walking is more limited by their shortness of breath is unlikely to benefit from revascularization. If risk factors are controlled, the rate of progression to critical limb ischemia (CLI) in claudicants is less than 10% per year in the first year after diagnosis, and lower in subsequent years [4]. Diabetes and lower ankle–brachial indices (ABIs) are associated with an increased risk of progression to rest pain and these patients, in particular, should be closely followed [5].

Given that revascularization for claudication is solely to address the symptoms of PAD, the risks and benefits of any intervention must be carefully evaluated. The procedural risk must be balanced against the anticipated improvement in lower extremity symptoms, factoring in a realistic appraisal of the durability of the intervention. Risk factor reduction, smoking cessation, and a walking program may produce modest improvements in some patients, and traditionally were always the first step. Multiple trials have demonstrated that supervised walking and medical management can improve symptoms [6]. There is increasing evidence that an endovascular intervention along with a supervised exercise program may produce greater improvements in walking distance and quality of life [7, 8] than supervised exercise alone; however, this is not yet the standard of care.

When to Refer Patients with CLI

Patients with CLI should always be referred for revascularization. The Trans-Atlantic Society Consensus (TASC), a society consisting of representatives

---

Box 8.1   Critical limb ischemia as defined by the Trans-Atlantic Society Consensus (TASC). Symptoms should be present for > 2 weeks [9]

Symptoms

- Chronic ischemic rest pain *or*
- Ischemic skin changes (ulcerations or gangrene)

Confirmatory studies

- Ankle–brachial indices (ABIs)
- Toe pressures
- Transcutaneous oxygen saturations

---

from the major vascular surgery, cardiology, and interventional radiology societies, defines CLI as chronic ischemic rest pain or ischemic skin changes (ulcerations or gangrene) (Box 8.1). These must be present for > 2 weeks and should be confirmed by ABIs, toe pressures, or transcutaneous oxygen saturations. Rest pain most commonly occurs at an ankle pressure < 50 mmHg and a toe pressure < 30 mmHg [9] or tissue loss with pressures < 70 mmHg and < 50 mmHg, respectively.

Critical limb ischemia can also present acutely, or as an acute-on-chronic phenomenon. For diagnostic purposes, ischemia of less than 14 days' duration is considered acute limb ischemia. These patients are at higher risk for limb loss because they have not yet developed collaterals and should be referred emergently, as the risk for limb loss decreases the sooner they are able to undergo revscularization [10]. Table 8.2 shows Rutherford's classification of the viability of limbs with acute ischemia based on several physical examination findings [11]. Given the need for prompt intervention in order to facilitate limb salvage, in the setting of acute, or acute-on-chronic, limb ischemia, referral to the emergency department may be the most expedient option.

Table 8.2 Rutherford classification of acute limb ischemia. Physical examination findings at the time of presentation correlate with the viability of the limb and help to dictate management [11].

	Viable	Threatened	Non-viable
Pain	Mild	Severe	Variable
Capillary refill	Intact	Delayed	Absent
Motor deficit	None	Partial	Complete
Sensory deficit	None	Partial	Complete
Arterial Doppler	Audible	Inaudible	Inaudible
Venous Doppler	Audible	Audible	Inaudible

Patients with CLI are at much higher risk of limb loss than individuals who present with claudication. American College of Cardiology/American Heart Association (AHA/ACC) guidelines suggest that at 1 year, only 50% of patients with CLI are alive with two limbs; an estimated 25% will have died from a cardiovascular etiology, and the remaining 25% will have undergone a major amputation [12]. The decision to proceed with revascularization, however, must be made on an individual basis, in each case weighing the risks and benefits of the proposed procedure. In patents who have a limited life expectancy or a prohibitive perioperative risk, or who are non-ambulatory at baseline, the decision may be made to forgo limb salvage. A caveat is that in patients who are non-ambulatory due to a prior amputation, the remaining leg may, paradoxically, take on increased functional importance, allowing them to transfer and pivot independently. Futility must also be recognized in patients who have undergone multiple prior failed revascularizations and in whom further attempts are unlikely to yield successful or durable limb salvage. Once the decision has been made that revascularization is not going to be pursued, then decisions about treatment move to determining the level of amputation based on the likelihood of the amputation healing. Making these decisions requires experience, good judgment, and an ability to communicate well with the patent and family.

Revascularization Options and Results

Open, endovascular, and hybrid approaches to revascularization have all been described, and there is no universally correct approach that is suitable for all patients. Rather, each patient must be evaluated individually, taking into account the location and characteristics of the occlusive disease, the patient's overall health and comorbidities, and the availability of autogenous conduit. Consensus guidelines, such as those developed by TASC, robust clinical outcomes data, and practitioner experience provide guidance in selecting the correct therapy for each patient.

Iliac Revascularizations

The treatment of iliac disease can be acheived with either open or endovascular approaches. For disease of the lower portion of the aorta and bilateral iliac arteries, the anatomic distribution of the lesions should guide treatment. There are several systems of classification, but the most widely used is that developed by TASC (Figure 8.1) [9]. Endovascular modalities are the first-line treatment for TASC A and B lesions, and as technology has advanced, TASC C lesions can increasingly be treated with endovascular approaches. TASC D lesions are best treated with open surgical procedures. This is motivated by evidence attesting to the durability of iliac stents, with 71–82% of stents remaining patent at

Type A lesions

• Unilateral or bilateral stenoses of CIA
• Unilateral or bilateral single short (≤3 cm) stenosis of EIA

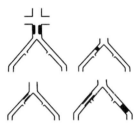

Type B lesions

• Short (≤3 cm) stenosis of infrarenal aorta
• Unilateral CIA occlusion
• Single or multiple stenosis totaling 3–10 cm involving the
  EIA not extending into the CFA
• Unilateral EIA occlusion not involving the origins of
  internal iliac or CFA

Type C lesions

• Bilateral CIA occlusions
• Bilateral EIA stenoses 3–10 cm long not extending into
  the CFA
• Unilateral EIA stenosis extending into the CFA
• Unilateral EIA occlusion that involves the origins of
  internal iliac and/or CFA
• Heavily calcified unilateral EIA occlusion with or without
  involvement of origins of internal iliac and/or CFA

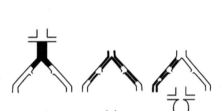

Type D lesions

• Infra-renal aorto-iliac occlusion
• Diffuse disease involving the aorta and both iliac arteries
  requiring treatment
• Diffuse multiple stenoses involving the unilateral CIA,
  EIA, and CFA
• Unilateral occlusions of both CIA and EIA
• Bilateral occlusions of EIA
• Iliac stenoses in patients with AAA requiring treatment
  and not amenable to endograft placement or other
  lesions requiring open aortic or iliac surgery

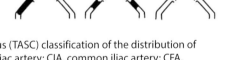

Figure 8.1 Trans-Atlantic Society Consensus (TASC) classification of the distribution of aorto-iliac occlusive disease. EIA, external iliac artery; CIA, common iliac artery; CFA, common femoral artery; AAA, abdominal aortic aneurysm. *Source*: adapted with permission from TASC paper [9].

2 years. A multicenter randomized trial comparing bare metal stents (BMS) with covered stents showed that they had similar patency for TASC A and B lesions, but that covered stents had superior patency for TASC C lesions [13, 14]

Open revascularization for aorto-iliac disease has a robust history and significant long-term follow-up data are available. These bypasses tend to remain patent and are very durable. Patency at 1 year is as high as 96%, which in the same series is accompanied by 71% patency at an impressive 15 years of follow-up [15]. As such, the gold standard for aorto-iliac revascularization is an aortobifemoral bypass graft using prosthetic conduit (Figure 8.2). This operation can be performed either via a midline incision and transperitoneal approach or via a flank incision and retroperitoneal approach.

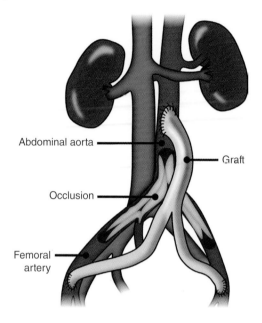

Abdominal aorta

Graft

Occlusion

Femoral
artery

Figure 8.2 Aortobifemoral bypass.

An aortobifemoral bypass is not a trivial undertaking; however, the peri-operative morbidity and mortality are acceptable with careful patient selection. A meta-analysis that included patients dating back to the 1970s showed a mortality rate of 4.1% and a 5-year patency of 86% [16]. As with all vascular procedures, there is a risk of complications related to underlying patient disease as well as complications related to the graft.

An aortobifemoral bypass is a major vascular operation, and anatomic factors such as previous abdominal operations, large ventral hernias, the presence of a colostomy or urostomy, or a prior failed aortobifemoral bypass may make extra-anatomic bypass operations a more attractive option. The most common of these operations is an axillobifemoral bypass, although other configurations have been described (Figure 8.3) This bypass can be performed using either the right or the left axillary artery as the source of inflow, provided there is no atherosclerotic disease or significant stenosis. A prosthetic graft is tunneled under the skin along the flank and anastomosed to the femoral artery on one side; a femoral-femoral crossover bypass is then performed to bring blood to the other leg. In mixed populations of patients with claudication and CLI, primary patency at 5 years ranges from 58% to 78% [17, 18]. Procedure-specific complications include injury to structures near the axillary artery, such as the brachial plexus, as well as risk of embolism to the arm as a consequence of clamping the axillary artery.

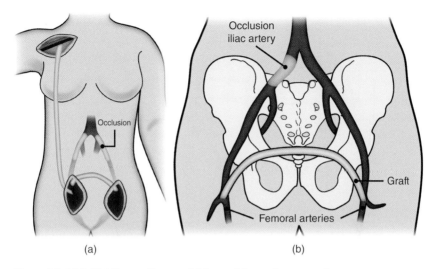

Figure 8.3 (a) Axillobifemoral bypass; (b) femoral-femoral crossover bypass.

In the circumstances where there is unilateral iliac disease, aorto-iliac and femoral-femoral crossover bypass procedures have excellent results. Femoral-femoral crossover bypass procedures can also be employed in hybrid operations with unilateral iliac stenting. The femoral-femoral bypass itself has excellent patency, estimated to be 75% at 5 years [9]. In this bypass, a prosthetic graft is sewn to both femoral arteries and tunneled just above the pubic symphysis. In instances of infection, or infected fields, vein can be used; however, prosthetic material is more commonly employed for this bypass. Aorto-iliac bypasses have been shown to have a lower patency rate than aortofemoral bypasses [19], so this option is generally reserved for patients where a groin incision would ideally be avoided, such as those with multiple prior groin operations or groin radiation.

Non-bypass options for revascularization, such as aorto-iliac endarterectomy, have historically demonstrated good results. In the current era, this procedure has taken on a more limited role. In general, it is best employed in individuals with heavily calcified focal lesions of the aorta and proximal iliac arteries. The operation involves accessing the aorta in an open fashion, either through the midline or a flank incision, and removing the portion of plaque causing the stenosis. It can be performed without the use of prosthetic material, which is useful in an infected field. As it has fallen out of favor, results in the literature are scant, but those that are reported show patency of up to 89% at 10 years [20].

Femoropopliteal Disease

Disease in the femoropopliteal location most often involves the superficial femoral artery (SFA) [21]. There have been significant advances in the

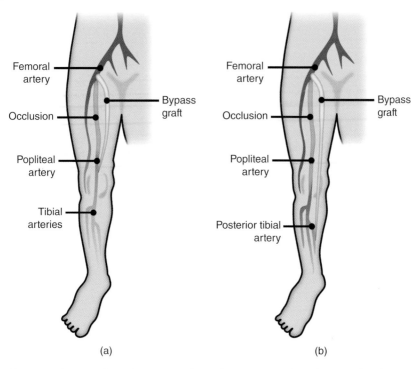

Figure 8.4 Bypasses from the common femoral artery to: (a) above-knee popliteal artery; (b) posterior tibial artery.

endovascular treatment of SFA disease, including the use of covered and drug-eluting stents, drug-eluting balloons, and a wide range of atherectomy devices. Despite this, surgical revascularization with bypasses such as those from the common femoral artery to the above- or below-knee popliteal artery (Figure 8.4) remain the gold-standard approach, with reported patency as high as 88% at 3 years for femoropopliteal bypass grafts with vein [22].

Although there have been significant advances since it was last revised, the TASC II recommendations offer guidance as to which types of lesion may best be initially approached using open surgical bypass [9]. Table 8.3 and Figure 8.5 show the classification of femoropopliteal disease according to the TASC II guidelines. Society recommendations are that TASC A lesions be treated with endovascular therapy, and TASC D lesions undergo open surgical revascularization. TASC B and C lesions can be treated by either open or endovascular methods, depending on factors such as patient comorbidities and anatomy, surgeon experience, and the availability of endovascular resources.

When planning a surgical bypass, the choice of conduit is among the largest determinants of long-term outcomes. The patient's own vein, typically the

Table 8.3 Trans-Atlantic Inter-Society Consensus (TASC II) classification of femoropopliteal disease [9].

Type	Lesion characteristics
A	Single stenosis ≤ 10 cm
	Single occlusion ≤ 5 cm
B	Multiple stenosis or occlusions, each ≤ 5 cm
	Single stenosis or occlusion ≤ 15 cm not involving infrageniculate popliteal artery
	Single or multiple lesions in the absence of continuous tibial vessels to improve inflow for tibial bypass
	Heavily calcified occlusion ≤ 5 cm
	Single popliteal stenosis
C	Multiple stenoses or occlusions totaling > 15 cm with or without heavy calcification
	Recurrent stenoses or occlusions that need treatment after two endovascular interventions
D	Chronic occlusion of common or superficial femoral artery > 20 cm or involving popliteal artery
	Chronic occlusion of popliteal artery and proximal trifurcation vessels

ipsilateral greater saphenous vein, is near-universally agreed upon as providing the best long-term patency for all bypass grafts below the inguinal ligament [23]. Additionally, bypasses to the above-knee popliteal artery have better patency than those to the below-knee popliteal artery. A large meta-analysis of such grafts when performed with vein showed a 5-year patency of 77% for vein grafts to the above-knee popliteal artery, but 65% to the below-knee popliteal artery; however, both patency rates are acceptable and likely to provide significant benefit to patients [24].

In the absence of available autogenous conduit, prosthetic may be used. The long-term patency rates with prosthetic bypasses vary based on the extent of the bypass. In addition to the traditional options of Dacron or polytetrafluoroethylene (PTFE), newer grafts, including those bonded to heparin, have become available. Patency with heparin-bonded grafts is generally better than traditional PTFE, with rates reported to be as high as 86% at 1 year in femoral to above-knee popliteal bypass grafts [25]. The use of antiplatelet agents, such as aspirin and clopidogrel, have been shown to increase patency in peripheral bypass grafts [26], especially those to the below-knee popliteal artery.

Tibioperoneal Disease

Disease in the peroneal and the anterior and posterior tibial arteries is often seen in diabetic patients. Interventions for the tibial arteries are generally

Type A lesions

• Single stenosis ≤ 10 cm in length
• Single occlusion ≤ 5 cm in length

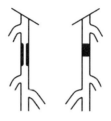

Type B lesions

• Multiple lesions (stenoses or occlusions), each ≤ 5 cm
• Single stenosis or occlusion ≤ 15 cm not involving the infrageniculate popliteal artery
• Single or multiple lesions in the absence of continuous tibial vessels to improve inflow for a distal bypass
• Heavily calcified occlusion ≤ 5 cm in length
• Single popliteal stenosis

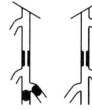

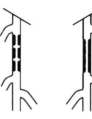

Type C lesions

• Multiple stenoses or occlusions totaling > 15 cm with or without heavy calcification
• Recurrent stenoses or occlusions that need treatment after two endovascular interventions

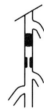

Type D lesions

• Chronic total occlusions of CFA or SFA (> 20 cm, involving the popliteal artery)
• Chronic total occlusion of popliteal artery and proximal trifurcation vessels

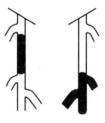

Figure 8.5 Trans-Atlantic Society Consensus (TASC) classification of the distribution of femoropopliteal occlusive disease. CFA, common femoral artery; SFA, superficial femoral artery. *Source*: adapted with permission from TASC paper [9].

restricted to individuals with rest pain or tissue loss. Although tibial angioplasty is gaining in popularity and may be appropriate in some settings, an open bypass to a target below the knee or even the foot may be necessary to provide adequate blood flow. As with all bypasses, the long-term patency is determined by the adequacy of the inflow, the conduit, and the outflow.

The proximal site of the bypass is frequently dictated by the amount of available conduit. The site of the proximal bypass does not influence the patency of the bypass [27, 28], although it is important to make sure that there is no significant disease in the inflow vessels. In some circumstances, a hybrid approach of using endovascular options to treat the inflow and then a surgical bypass as outflow are most appropriate [29]. An example of this would be a stent placed in the SFA above a bypass from the above-knee popliteal artery to the dorsalis pedis artery in a patient with a foot ulcer and minimal autogenous vein to use a conduit.

As in bypasses above the knee, vein is the preferred conduit, and its effect on patency for targets below the knee is even more pronounced. Primary patency rates for bypasses with prosthetic to the tibial arteries are as low as 30–39% at 3 years [30, 31]. Despite low primary patency rates, limb salvage can still be accomplished in a proportion of patients if the tissue loss can heal prior to the bypass occluding. In fact, the same studies reporting primary patency of 30–39% also reported limb salvage of 61–71% at 1 year in the same patients [30, 31]. Depending on the specific anatomy of the patient, the patency rates with a prosthetic bypass may be low enough to render the operation futile; this is a decision best made by a specialist. In general, diffuse disease in the tibial arteries predicts poor patency rates.

Below the knee, several technical considerations have been attempted to improve the overall poor patency with prosthetic. A cuff of vein can be sewn between the distal end of the prosthetic and the distal target vessel. There are various configurations of vein cuffs, a detailed discussion of which is beyond the scope of this chapter. Multiple small studies have been performed on the use of these, and meta-analyses have shown that they improve primary patency [32] as well as limb salvage [33], although large randomized controlled trials have not been performed. The intentional creation of arteriovenous fistulas to improve outflow can also augment limb salvage rates [34].

In some patients with CLI, diffuse tibial disease gives way to patent vessels within the foot. In selected circumstances, bypasses can be performed from the below-knee popliteal artery or tibial arteries themselves to patent vessels in the foot. These cases can only be performed if there is adequate vein, as prosthetic grafts do not have acceptable patency rates. Series from select centers report primary patency as high as 58–80% at 1 year, with an accompanying limb salvage rate of 77–90% [35, 36].

Complications of Revascularization

Complications of revascularization include both systemic and local complications. Patients with vascular disease typically have multiple comorbidities, and therefore complications must not be taken lightly.

Cardiac complications are a major cause of morbidity and mortality in patients undergoing open revascularization given their overwhelming burden of atherosclerotic disease. Myocardial infarction occurs in 2.3–14% of patients undergoing peripheral vascular procedures [37, 38]. Routine screening for cardiac disease as well as preoperative cardiac optimization is recommended. Peri-operative beta-blockade should be continued postoperatively in patients who have an indication for it, but evidence is equivocal as to whether beta-blockade should be started on all vascular patients prior to undergoing vascular surgery [39, 40].

Respiratory complications following vascular procedures are more common in patients undergoing thoracic procedures or who have a history of smoking. Complications include atelectasis and pneumonia. Prevention, including pre-operative optimization and aggressive pulmonary toilet postoperatively, is crucial. The importance of smoking cessation cannot be overemphasized.

Renal failure can also occur following a vascular procedure. This is most often due to acute tubular necrosis, either from ischemic injury in the case of an aortic clamp above the renal arteries, atheroemboli, or toxic injury from contrast dye. Acute tubular necrosis due to contrast dye can be prevented with hydration pre- and postoperatively, with either normal saline or a sodium bicarbonate infusion. An elevated creatinine preoperatively increases the risk of kidney injury, but pre-existing chronic kidney disease is not prohibitive for most procedures. Mannitol may be used to minimize oliguric uremia in aortic operations.

Graft thrombosis is one of the leading local complications follow open revascularizations. The etiology of graft thrombosis following bypass varies based on its timing following surgery. Early graft thrombosis is most often due to a technical issue, and should be addressed immediately with thrombectomy of the graft and revision of any technical problems. If no technical issues are discovered, patients are most often anticoagulated, and a hypercoagulable work-up is performed postoperatively. Graft thrombosis within the first 2 years but out of the immediate postoperative period is most often due to neointimal hyperplasia. To treat thrombosis after the immediate postoperative period, grafts may be thrombectomized and an angiogram performed to determine any areas of stenosis. Further open or endovascular treatment then depends on the angiogram findings. Graft thrombosis after 2 years is most often due to progression of the underlying disease.

Graft infection is a rarer but more dreaded complication. It occurs in 1–5% of grafts [24, 41] and may require complete removal of the graft, especially if it is a prosthetic conduit. *Staphylococcus epidermidis* and methicillin-sensitive *Staphylococcus aureus* are the most common pathogens isolated [41], although other causative pathogens can include more virulent organisms, such as methicillin-resistant *Staphylococcus aureus* (MRSA). In the case of an infected prosthetic bypass, an extra-anatomic bypass may be required in addition to removal of the prior bypass in order to stay out of the infected field. This is ideally performed with vein, although alternatives include rifampin-soaked prosthetic, antibiotic beads, or cadaveric homograft if vein is not available.

Anastomotic aneurysms can occur at either the proximal or distal anastomosis of a bypass graft. These are due to native arterial degeneration, infection, or mechanical stress. If these are small, they may be observed. If they are large, repair is mandatory due to the risk of rupture. The most pressing concern in the case of an anastomotic aneurysm is whether it occurred due to infection, particularly if there is any prosthetic within the operative field.

Aortic surgery carries its own unique set of complications. An aorto-enteric fistula is a rare entity, occurring in < 2% of all aortic operations [42], but it is a dramatic complication with a high rate of mortality. It most often occurs at the distal duodenum. Patients may have a herald bleed followed by exsanguination. The treatment is graft removal and extra-anatomic bypass or an *in situ* bypass with rifampin-soaked prosthetic or a cadaveric homograft. The affected intestine must also be removed. A less dramatic but also distressing complication of aortic surgery is erectile dysfunction due to lack of blood flow to the internal iliac arteries. Disruption of per-aortic nerve fibers can also produce retrograde ejaculation.

Preoperative Evaluation and Management

The biggest concern in patients with PAD is their risk of cardiac complications. According to joint guidelines from the AHA/ACC [43], the combination of the surgical procedure and the individual patient's clinical risk factors dictate what, if any, formal cardiac testing they should undergo prior to their planned intervention. In general, for higher-risk procedures, pharmacologic cardiac stress testing may be recommended if a patient's functional capacity is difficult to determine. This is often the case in vascular patients whose ability to ambulate is limited by the very disease for which they seek treatment.

The fundamentals of medical therapy should not be overlooked as part of the per-operative preparation for an open or endovascular procedure. Smoking cessation improves outcomes and reduces the risk of long-term complications. Blood glucose control is important in patients with concomitant diabetes. Management of hypertension and hyperlipidemia is also important in this population with their high burden of comorbidities.

Conclusion

Patients with peripheral vascular disease tend to have a high burden of comorbidities and depending on the exact nature of their PAD, may benefit the most from an open or endovascular procedure, or simply medical management. Referral to a specialist for symptomatic patients can help to determine the best course of action and confirm the diagnosis.

References

1 Fontaine R, Kim M, Kieny R. [Surgical treatment of peripheral circulation disorders]. Helv Chir Acta. 1954; 21: 499–533.

2 McGrae McDermott M, Mehta S, *et al.* Exertional leg symptoms other than intermittent claudication are common in peripheral arterial disease. Arch Intern Med. 1999; 159: 387.

3 Conte MS, Pomposelli FB, Clair DG, *et al.* Society for Vascular Surgery practice guidelines for atherosclerotic occlusive disease of the lower extremities: Management of asymptomatic disease and claudication. J Vasc Surg. 2015; 61: 2S–41S.

4 Dormandy J, Heeck L, Vig S. The natural history of claudication: risk to life and limb. Semin Vasc Surg. 1999; 12: 123–37.

5 Aquino R, Johnnides C, Makaroun M, *et al.* Natural history of claudication: Long-term serial follow-up study of 1244 claudicants. J Vasc Surg. 2001; 34: 962–970.

6 Lane R, Ellis B, Watson L, *et al.* Exercise for intermittent claudication. In: Lane R, ed. Cochrane Database of Systematic Reviews. Chichester, UK: John Wiley & Sons, Ltd. Epub ahead of print 18 July 2014. DOI: 10.1002/14651858. CD000990.pub3.

7 Fakhry F, Spronk S, van der Laan L, *et al.* Endovascular revascularization and supervised exercise for peripheral artery disease and intermittent claudication. JAMA. 2015; 314: 1936.

8 Frans FA, Bipat S, Reekers JA, *et al.* Systematic review of exercise training or percutaneous transluminal angioplasty for intermittent claudication. Br J Surg. 2012; 99: 16–28.

9 Norgren L, Hiatt WR, Dormandy JA, *et al.* Inter-Society Consensus for the Management of Peripheral Arterial Disease (TASC II). J Vasc Surg. 2007; 45: S5-67.

10 Stile T. Results of a prospective randomized trial evaluating surgery versus thrombolysis for ischemia of the lower extremity. The STILE trial. Ann Surg. 1994; 220: 251–66.

11 Rutherford RB, Flanigan DP, Gupta SK, *et al.* Suggested standards for reports dealing with lower extremity ischemia. J Vasc Surg. 1986; 4: 80–94.

12 Hirsch AT, Haskal ZJ, Hertzer NR, *et al.* ACC/AHA 2005 Practice Guidelines for the Management of Patients With Peripheral Arterial Disease (Lower Extremity, Renal, Mesenteric, and Abdominal Aortic). Circulation 2006; 113: e463–465.

13 Mwipatayi BP, Thomas S, Wong J, *et al.* A comparison of covered vs bare expandable stents for the treatment of aortoiliac occlusive disease. J Vasc Surg. 2011; 54: 1561–70.

14 Mwipatayi BP, Sharma S, Daneshmand A, *et al.* Durability of the balloon-expandable covered versus bare-metal stents in the Covered versus Balloon Expandable Stent Trial (COBEST) for the treatment of aortoiliac occlusive disease. J Vasc Surg. 2016; 64: 83–94.e1.

15 Hertzer NR, Bena JF, Karafa MT. A personal experience with direct reconstruction and extra-anatomic bypass for aortoiliofemoral occlusive disease. J Vasc Surg. 2007; 45: 527–535.e3.

16 Chiu KWH, Davies RSM, Nightingale PG, *et al*. Review of direct anatomical open surgical management of atherosclerotic aorto-iliac occlusive disease. Eur J Vasc Endovasc Surg. 2010; 39: 460–71.

17 Liedenbaum MH, Verdam FJ, Spelt D, *et al*. The outcome of the axillofemoral bypass: a retrospective analysis of 45 patients. World J Surg. 2009; 33: 2490–6.

18 El-Massry S, Saad E, Sauvage LR, *et al*. Axillofemoral bypass with externally supported, knitted Dacron grafts: A follow-up through twelve years. J Vasc Surg. 1993; 17: 107–115.

19 Baird RJ, Feldman P, Miles JT, *et al*. Subsequent downstream repair after aorta-iliac and aorta-femoral bypass operations. Surgery. 1977; 82: 785–93.

20 Connolly JE, Price T. Aortoiliac endarterectomy: a lost art? Ann Vasc Surg 2006; 20: 56–62.

21 Morris-Stiff G, Ogunbiyi S, Rees J, *et al*. Variations in the anatomical distribution of peripheral vascular disease according to gender. Ann R Coll Surg Engl. 2011; 93: 306–9.

22 Watelet J, Cheysson E, Poels D, *et al*. In situ versus reversed saphenous vein for femoropopliteal bypass: a prospective randomized study of 100 cases. Ann Vasc Surg. 1987; 1: 441–52.

23 Twine CP, McLain AD. Graft type for femoro-popliteal bypass surgery. In: Twine CP, ed. Cochrane Database of Systematic Reviews. Chichester, UK: John Wiley & Sons, Ltd. Epub ahead of print 12 May 2010. DOI: 10.1002/14651858. CD001487.pub2.

24 Pereira CE, Albers M, Romiti M, *et al*. Meta-analysis of femoropopliteal bypass grafts for lower extremity arterial insufficiency. J Vasc Surg. 2006; 44: 510–517.e3.

25 Kirkwood ML, Wang GJ, Jackson BM, *et al*. Lower limb revascularization for PAD using a heparin-coated PTFE conduit. Vasc Endovascular Surg. 2011; 45: 329–34.

26 Bedenis R, Lethaby A, Maxwell H, *et al*. Antiplatelet agents for preventing thrombosis after peripheral arterial bypass surgery. Cochrane Database Syst Rev. Epub ahead of print 19 February 2015. DOI: 10.1002/14651858. CD000535.pub3.

27 Shibuya T, Shinntani T, Edogawa S, *et al*. Examination of Difference in the Proximal Anastomotic Site for Crus, Ankle Bypass: Common Femoral Artery vs Below the Knee Popliteal Artery. Ann Vasc Dis. 2012; 5: 30–5.

28 Veith FJ, Ascer E, Gupta SK, *et al*. Tibiotibial vein bypass grafts: a new operation for limb salvage. J Vasc Surg. 1985; 2: 552–7.

29 Wengerter KR, Yang PM, Veith FJ, *et al*. A twelve-year experience with the popliteal-to-distal artery bypass: The significance and management of proximal disease. J Vasc Surg. 1992; 15: 143–151.

30 Parsons RE, Suggs WD, Veith FJ, *et al*. Polytetrafluoroethylene bypasses to infrapopliteal arteries without cuffs or patches: a better option than amputation in patients without autologous vein. J Vasc Surg. 1996; 23 (2): 347–356.

31 Veith FJ, Gupta SK, Ascer E, *et al*. Six-year prospective multicenter randomized comparison of autologous saphenous vein and expanded polytctrafluoroethylene grafts in infrainguinal arterial reconstructions. J Vasc Surg. 1986; 3: 104–14.

32 Khalil AA, Boyd A, Griffiths G. Interposition vein cuff for infragenicular prosthetic bypass graft. In: Khalil AA, ed. Cochrane Database of Systematic Reviews. Chichester, UK: John Wiley & Sons, Ltd. Epub ahead of print 12 September 2012. DOI: 10.1002/14651858.CD007921.pub2.

33 Twine CP, Williams IM, Fligelstone LJ. Systematic review and meta-analysis of vein cuffs for below-knee synthetic bypass. Br J Surg. 2012; 99: 1195–202.

34 Kreienberg PB, Darling RC, Chang BB, *et al*. Adjunctive techniques to improve patency of distal prosthetic bypass grafts: Polytetrafluoroethylene with remote arteriovenous fistulae versus vein cuffs. J Vasc Surg. 2000; 31: 696–701.

35 Uhl C, Hock C, Betz T, *et al*. Pedal bypass surgery after crural endovascular intervention. J Vasc Surg. 2014; 59: 1583–7.

36 Pomposelli FB, Kansal N, Hamdan AD, *et al*. A decade of experience with dorsalis pedis artery bypass: Analysis of outcome in more than 1000 cases. J Vasc Surg. 2003; 37: 307–315.

37 McFalls EO, Ward HB, Moritz TE, *et al*. Coronary-artery revascularization before elective major vascular surgery. N Engl J Med. 2004; 351: 2795–2804.

38 Simons JP, Baril DT, Goodney PP, *et al*. The effect of postoperative myocardial ischemia on long-term survival after vascular surgery. J Vasc Surg. 2013; 58: 1600–8.

39 POISE Study Group, Devereaux PJ, Yang H, *et al*. Effects of extended-release metoprolol succinate in patients undergoing non-cardiac surgery (POISE trial): a randomised controlled trial. Lancet. 2008; 371: 1839–47.

40 Bouri S, Shun-Shin MJ, Cole GD, *et al*. Meta-analysis of secure randomised controlled trials of β-blockade to prevent perioperative death in non-cardiac surgery. Heart. 2014; 100: 456–64.

41 Siracuse JJ, Nandivada P, Giles KA, *et al*. Prosthetic graft infections involving the femoral artery. J Vasc Surg. 2013; 57: 700–5.

42 Busuttil SJ, Goldstone J. Diagnosis and management of aortoenteric fistulas. Semin Vasc Surg. 2001; 14: 302–11.

43 Fleisher LA, Fleischmann KE, Auerbach AD, *et al*. 2014 ACC/AHA guideline on perioperative cardiovascular evaluation and management of patients undergoing noncardiac surgery: a report of the American College of Cardiology/American Heart Association Task Force on practice guidelines. J Am Coll Cardiol. 2014; 64: e77–137.

Index

a
abdominal aortic aneurysm
        (AAA)   41, 48
    rupture   41
abdominal bruits   48–49
abdominal examination   48–49
abdominal pain   41–42
abnormal vascular reactivity   1
ACCF/AHA guidelines on endovascular
        treatment   131–132
acrocyanosis   45
acrogeria   46
acute limb ischemia (ALI)   2
    amputation rate   13
    definition   3
    mortality rate   13
    prevalence and incidence   13
    referral for surgical
            management   165
    symptoms (six Ps)   3, 44
Adson's maneuver   52
age-related incidence and prevalence of
        PAD   5–8
age, risk factor for PAD   13–14
alcohol intake, PAD risk and   19
Allen test and reverse Allen test   50
amaurosis fugax   38
amputation
    in acute limb ischemia   13
    in critical limb ischemia   12, 131

smoking risk factor in PAD   15
anemia   47
angiosomes   154–155
    of the foot and lower leg   135–136,
        138
angiotensin-converting enzyme (ACE)
        inhibitors   112, 113
angiotensin receptor blockers
        (ARB)   112, 113
ankle–brachial index (ABI)   37
    and segmental pressures   63–65
antiphospholipid antibodies, PAD risk
        and   19
antiphospholipid syndrome   45
antiplatelet agents, studies   116–117
anxiety, risk factor for PAD   19
aortic aneurysm   46
    chest examination   48
aortic dissection   40
aortic rupture   40
aortic surgery, risks related to   175
aortic valve regurgitation   40
aortobifemoral bypass   167–168
aorto-iliac bypass   169
aorto-iliac endarterectomy   169
aorto-iliac interventions   145–147
    angioplasty versus
            stenting   146–147
    PTFE-covered versus bare metal
            balloon-expandable stents   147

Peripheral Artery Disease, Second Edition. Edited by Emile R. Mohler and Michael R. Jaff.
© 2017 John Wiley & Sons Ltd. Published 2017 by John Wiley & Sons Ltd.

aorto-iliac PAD   119
aorto-iliac revascularization   167–169
arterial insufficiency
      assessment   51–52
arterial tortuosity   46
arterial ulcers   49
arterial ultrasound imaging   1–2
arteria lusoria   40
arterial wall dysplasia   1
arteriosclerosis obliterans   1
ascending aorta dissection   40
aspirin   116–117, 141, 143
asymptomatic PAD   2
   prevalence and incidence   8–10
atherectomy   152–153
atheromatous embolization   47
atherosclerosis   1
   development of   1–2
   eye examination   47
   risk factor for PAD   13
   risk factors   2
   subclinical   1–2
atherosclerotic risk factor medical
      management   111–117
   antiplatelet agents   116–117
   diabetes mellitus   113–114
   hyperlipidemia   114
   hypertension   112–113
   smoking cessation   114–116
atypical leg pain
   definition   2–3
   prevalence and incidence   12
auscultation
   for bruits   52–53
   carotid artery   47
awareness of PAD in the
      community   20–21
axillobifemoral bypass   168–169

b
bare metal balloon-expandable
      stents   147
Behçet's disease   50

beta-blockers   112
bivalirudin   140–141
blood pressure   46
   medical management   112–113
blood pressure measurement, history
      of   58–59
BMI, and PAD risk   14, 17–18
bowel infarction   41
bruit occlusion test   53
bruits
   abdominal   48–49
   auscultation for   52–53
   detection of   47–48
Buerger's disease   49–50, 115
Buerger's test   51
bupropion   115
bypass operations, PAD risk and   19

c
cadmium, serum levels and PAD risk   19
calcium channel blockers   113
capillary refill test   51
cardiovascular accidents   38–39
cardiovascular disease, risk factor for
      PAD   14
carotid arterial pulse   47
carotid artery bruits   47, 52
carotid intimal medial
      thickness   1–2, 68
central cyanosis   46
cephalic index   46
cerebrovascular disease risk in
      PAD   111–112
chest examination   48
chest veins, dilated   46
chilblains   45
cholesterol deposits in arteries   1–2
cholesterol levels
   high cholesterol and PAD risk   14
   risk factors for PAD   15–16
   statin therapy   114
chronic exertional compartment
      syndrome   96, 103

chronic kidney disease (CKD)   113
    risk factor for PAD   19
cilostazol   118–120
classifications of PAD   42
claudication   42–44
    classification systems   130
    comparison of management
        strategies   119–120
    definition   2
    hallmark symptom of PAD   2
    pharmacotherapy   118
    prevalence and incidence   10–11
    when to refer for surgical
        management   163–164
cleft palate   46
clinical syndromes of PAD   2–3
clopidogrel   116–117, 141, 143
color flow scans   68–69
community awareness of
    PAD   20–21
computed tomography
        angiography   73–77
    advantages   76
    anaphylaxis   77
    artifacts   76
    basics   73–74
    calcification   76
    contrast-induced
        nephropathy   76–77
    image acquisition and
        interpretation   74–75
    pitfalls   76
    protocol   74–75
    radiation exposure   76
contrast-induced nephropathy   82
conventional angiography   81–84
    advantages   82
    allergic reactions   81, 82
    anaphylaxis   81, 82
    artifacts   84
    basics   81
    digital subtraction angiography
        (DSA)   82–83

image acquisition and
        interpretation   81–83
    informed consent   81
    limitations   84
    nephrogenic systemic fibrosis   82
    pitfalls   82–84
    pre-procedure patient care   81
    protocol   81–82
corneal arcus   46
coronary artery disease (CAD) risk in
        PAD   111–112
costoclavicular maneuver   52
cough   40
covered stents in femoropopliteal
        disease   151–152
C-reactive protein (CRP), risk factor
        for PAD   13, 14, 17
critical limb ischemia (CLI)   2, 44
    ACCF/AHA guidelines on
        endovascular
        treatment   131–132
    amputation risk   12, 131
    classification systems   130
    definition   3
    endovascular treatment   131–132
    indications for endovascular
        therapy   131
    limb prognosis   131
    lower extremity wound
        care   120–121
    overall survival   131
    patency issues   131
    prevalence and incidence   12–13
    typical anatomy in patients with
        CLI   131
    when to refer for surgical
        management   164–166
cryoplasty   153
cutaneous vasculitis   50
cutis marmorata   45
cutting balloon angioplasty   153
cystic adventitial disease   96,
        100–101

d

D-dimer, association with PAD   17
deep vein thrombophlebitis   49–50
depression, risk factor for PAD   19
diabetes mellitus
    eye examination   47
    medical management   113–114
    risk factor for atherosclerosis   2
    risk factor for PAD   13, 14, 15
diagnostic approach, patients with leg
    pain on exertion   104
Dieter test   39
differential diagnosis for PAD   92–94
digital subtraction angiography
    (DSA)   82–83
digit ischemia   49–50
dolichocephaly   46
Doppler combined with 2D imaging
    (duplex scanning)   68–69
Doppler ultrasound devices
    functions   59
    motion detection   59
    waveform analysis   60
drug-coated balloon (DCB) therapy in
    femoropopliteal
    disease   150–151
drug-eluting stents in femoropopliteal
    arteries   149–150
duplex scanning   67–69
    background and history   67
    color flow scans   68–69
    Doppler (hemodynamic)   68–69
    imaging (anatomy)   67–68
dyslipidemia, risk factor for
    PAD   15–16
dysphagia   40, 41
    aortica   40
    lusoria   40
dyspnea   40–41

e

ectopia lentis   46, 47
Ehlers–Danlos syndrome   46

type IV   100
electronic cigarettes   115–116
embolus   44
enalapril   112
endovascular treatment of
    PAD   129–156
    access   138–139
    anticoagulation   139–141
    antiplatelet
        management   141–143
    aorto-iliac interventions   145–147
    background for endovascular
        therapy   132–144
    chronic total occlusions   143–144
    clinical background   129–132
    clinical evidence for peripheral
        intervention   145–155
    critical limb ischemia   131–132
    femoropopliteal
        interventions   147–153
    history of development   129
    indications for   129
    intermittent
        claudication   129–131
    pedal interventions   153–155
    peripheral arterial
        anatomy   132–136
    post-procedural care   155
    pre-procedural imaging   136–138
    radiation   143
    re-entry devices   143–144
    technical background   136–144
    tibioperoneal
        interventions   153–155
    vascular angiosomes of the foot and
        lower leg   135–136, 138
end-stage PAD   44
enophthalmos   46
epidemiology of PAD   1–26
erectile dysfunction, complication of
    aortic surgery   175
ethnicity, PAD prevalence related
    to   3–6

everolimus-eluting self-expanding nitinol stent 149–150
exercise testing in the vascular laboratory 64–65
exercise therapy 118–119
exertional compartment syndrome 96, 103
external iliac artery endofibrosis (EIAE) 96, 98–99
extremity pain, symptom analysis 42–44
eyes, examination 46, 47

f
facial plethora 46
family history of PAD, risk factor for PAD 19–20
fatty streaks, development in arteries 1–2
femoral artery bruits 52–53
femoral–femoral crossover bypass 168–169
femoropopliteal disease, TASC II classification 147–148
femoropopliteal interventions 147–153
angioplasty versus stenting 149
atherectomy 152–153
covered stents 151–152
drug-coated balloon (DCB) therapy 150–151
drug-eluting stents in femoropopliteal arteries 149–150
specialty balloons 153
surgical revascularization 169–171, 172
TASC II classification of femoropopliteal PAD 147–148
fenofibrate 114
fetuin-A, PAD risk and 19
fibric acid derivatives 114

fibrinogen, risk factor for PAD 17
fibromuscular dysplasia 96, 99–100
Fontaine classification
claudication and critical limb ischemia 130
peripheral artery disease 42
foot
examination 49–50
ulcers 49

g
gangrene 3, 44, 120
genetic factors in PAD risk 19–20
glycoprotein IIb/IIIa receptor inhibitors 141

h
head and neck examination 46–48
heart failure 40
hemoptysis 40
hereditary hemorrhagic telangiectasia 46
high-density lipoprotein (HDL)-cholesterol 2, 14
high-income countries (HICs)
PAD risk factors 13–14
prevalence and incidence of PAD 3–5
hoarseness 41
Hollenhorst plaques 47
homocysteinemia, risk factor for PAD 13, 16–17
hyperabduction test 51–52
hypercholesterolemia, risk factor for PAD 15–16, 46
hyperhomocysteinemia, risk factor for PAD 13, 16–17
hyperinsulinemia, risk factor for PAD 15
hyperlipidemia
medical management 114
risk factor for PAD 13
hypertelorism 46

hypertension
  eye examination   47
  medical management   112–113
  risk factor for atherosclerosis   2
  risk factor for PAD   13, 14, 16
hypertriglyceridemia, and PAD   16
hypothenar hammer syndrome   45
hypothyroidism, PAD risk and   18

i
idiopathic mid-aortic syndrome   102
iliac revascularizations   166–169
imaging of PAD   73–87
  aorto-iliac
    CTA   85–86
    MRA   86
  computed tomography angiography
    (CTA)   73–77
  conventional angiography   81–84
  intravascular ultrasonography
    (IVUS)   84–85
  magnetic resonance angiography
    (MRA)   77–81
  pedal
    CTA   87
    MRA   87
  results from different imaging
    modalities   85–87
  runoff
    CTA   86, 87
    MRA   86–87
immunoglobulin-4 (IgG4)-related
  disease   41
incidence of PAD   3–13
inflammation   1, 17
inflammatory AAA   41
insulin resistance, risk factor for
  PAD   15
interleukin-6 (IL-6), association with
  PAD   17
intermittent claudication, endovascular
  treatment   129–131
intestinal angina   42

intravascular ultrasonography
  (IVUS)   84–85
  advantages   85
  basics   84
  pitfalls   85
ischemic rest pain   3, 44
ischemic stroke   38–39
ischemic ulcers   49

l
laser atherectomy   153
laser Doppler assessment of tissue
  perfusion   65–66
lead, serum levels and PAD risk   19
leg pain with exertion, diagnostic
  approach   104
limb ischemia   40
limb paresthesia and weakness   40
lips, blue   46
livedo racemosa   45
livedo reticularis   45
Loeys–Dietz syndrome   46
low-molecular-weight heparins   140
low-to middle-income countries
  (LMICs)
  PAD risk factors   13–14
  prevalence and incidence of
    PAD   3–5
lower extremities
  examination   49–50
  wound care   120–121
lower extremity arterial disease
  (LEAD)   1
lower extremity atherosclerotic
  PAD   1–2

m
magnetic resonance angiography
  (MRA)   77–81
  advantages   78, 80
  artifacts   80
  basics   77
  bolus timing   80

contrast enhanced MRA (CE-MRA) 78, 79
contrast-related nephrogenic systemic fibrosis 80
image acquisition and interpretation 77–78, 79
nephrogenic systemic fibrosis 80
non-contrast-enhanced MRA 77–78
patient claustrophobia in the MRI machine 80–81
patient motion problem 81
pitfalls 80–81
post-processing and interpretation 78
protocol 77
time-of-flight (TOF) angiography 77–78
time required 80
Marfan syndrome 46, 47, 48, 100
Medical Outcomes Study 12-item Short Form 119–120
medical therapy of PAD 111–121
aims 111
atherosclerotic risk factor management 111–117
comparison of claudication management strategies 119–120
exercise therapy 118–119
lower extremity wound care 120–121
management of claudication 117–119
mesenteric infarction 41–42
mesenteric ischemia 40, 41–42
mesenteric vein thrombosis 42
methicillin-resistant *Staphyllococcus aureus* (MRSA) graft infection 174
methotrexate 101
mortality rate for acute limb ischemia (ALI) 13

musculoskeletal pathology, and leg pain on exertion 96, 103–104
myocardial ischemia and infarction 40

n
natural history of PAD 22–24, 25
nausea and vomiting 42
neck distension 46
neck examination *see* head and neck examination
nephrogenic systemic fibrosis 80
neurologic symptoms of PAD 38–39
neuropathic ulcers 49
niacin 114
nicotine replacement therapy (NRT) 115
nisoldipine 112
non-atherosclerotic peripheral artery disease (NAPAD)
definition 91–92
diagnostic evaluation of patients with leg pain on exertion 104
differentiation from PAD 92–94
entities that make up NAPAD 94–104
presentation of PAD 91–92
treatment considerations 105
treatment of 96
when it should be suspected 92–94
non-HDL-cholesterol 2
non-healing ulcer 3

o
obesity
risk factor for atherosclerosis 2
risk factor for PAD 14, 17–18
oral health, poor, association with PAD 19
Osler–Weber–Rendu syndrome 46
outcomes of PAD 22–24, 25

p

paclitaxel-coated angioplasty
balloons 150–151
paclitaxel-coated Zilver stent 150
palpating for pulses 50–52
palpebral fissures, downward
sloping 46
pectus carinatum 48
pectus excavatum 48
pedal endovascular
interventions 153–155
pentoxifylline 118
percutaneous transluminal angioplasty
(PTA) 141, 143
peripheral artery disease (PAD)
clinical syndromes 2–3
definition 1–2
detection of clinical PAD 2
peripheral artery occlusive disease
(PAOD) 1
Peripheral Artery
Questionnaire 119
peripheral vascular disease (PVD) 1
pernio (chilblains) 45
photoplethysmograph (PPG) 65–66
physical activity, PAD risk and 19
physical examination 46–53
abdomen 48–49
arterial insufficiency
assessment 51–52
auscultation 52–53
blood pressure 46
chest 48
general appearance 46
head and neck
examination 46–48
lower extremity
examination 49–50
palpating for pulses 50–52
physiological testing 58–66
ankle–brachial index (ABI) and
segmental pressures 63–65
background and history 58–59

Doppler ultrasound
devices 59–60
establishment of the non-invasive
vascular laboratory 59
exercise testing 64–65
history of blood pressure
measurement 58–59
physiological invasive testing 58
physiological non-invasive
testing 58–59
plethysmography 58–59, 60–62
sphygmomanometry 59
tissue perfusion 65–66
transcutaneous oximetry
($TcPO_2$) 66
plaque formation 2
plaque rupture 1
plethysmography 58–59, 60–62
polytetrafluoroethylene (PTFE)-
covered stents 147
popliteal artery aneurysm
(PAA) 51
popliteal artery entrapment syndrome
(PAES) 94–98
population risk score for PAD 20
prasugrel 117
premature lower extremity
atherosclerosis (PLEA) 92, 94
presentation of PAD 91–92
prevalence of PAD 3–13, 37–38
population risk score 20
progression of PAD 20–22
pseudoxanthoma elasticum, arterial
manifestations 102–103
pulse detection,
plethysmography 60–62
pulses, palpating for 50–52
pulse volume recording (PVR)
amplitude 61
contour 62

q

quality-of-life questionnaires 119

r

race
  influence on PAD risk   18–19
  and PAD prevalence   3–6
radiating cardiac murmurs   47
ramipril   112
Raynaud phenomenon (RP)   45
re-entry devices for endovascular
    intervention   143–144
regional symptom analysis
  abdominal pain   41–42
  extremity pain   42–44
  neurologic symptoms   38–39
  skin manifestations   44–45
  thoracic symptoms   40–41
retrognathia   46
risk factors for atherosclerosis   2
risk factors for development of
    PAD   13–20
risk of PAD, identifying at-risk
    individuals   37–38
risk score for PAD prevalence in a
    population   20
Rutherford classification
  acute limb ischemia   165
  claudication and critical limb
      ischemia   130
  peripheral artery disease   42

s

sciatic artery, persistent   50
sclera, blue   46
scleroderma   45, 46
scoring balloon angioplasty   153
sex-based incidence and prevalence of
    PAD   5–8
sex-based risk of PAD   14
simvastatin   114
sirolimus-eluting self-expanding nitinol
    stent   149
skin manifestations of PAD   44–45
skin ulcers   44
smoking

risk factor for atherosclerosis   2
risk factor for PAD   13–15, 38
smoking cessation
  effects on risk of PAD   14–15
  studies   114–116
socioeconomic status, PAD risk
    and   19
solid bolus dysphagia   40
specialty balloons   153
sphygmomanometry   59
stage classifications of PAD   42
Staphylococcus epidermidis graft
    infection   174
statin therapy   114
stenting   119 *see also specific types of
    stent*
stridor   40
stroke   38–39
  and carotid bruits   47
subclavian steal   39
superficial thrombophlebitis   49–50
superior vena cava syndrome   41, 46
surgical management of
    PAD   163–175
  anastomotic aneurysms   175
  cardiac complications   173–174
  complications of
      revascularization   173–175
  erectile dysfunction
      complication   175
  femoropopliteal disease   169–171,
      172
  graft infection   174
  graft thrombosis   174
  iliac revascularizations   166–169
  preoperative patient evaluation and
      management   175
  referral of patients with acute limb
      ischemia   165
  renal failure risk   174
  respiratory complications   174
  revascularization options and
      results   166–173

surgical management of PAD (*contd.*)
  risks relating to aortic
    surgery 175
  tibioperoneal disease 171–173
  when to refer patients with
    claudication 163–164
  when to refer patients with
    CLI 164–166
symptoms *see* regional symptom
  analysis
systemic atherosclerosis, risk factor for
  PAD 13
systemic lupus erythematosus 45

t
Takayasu's arteritis 101–102
telangiectasia 46
telmisartan 112
temporal arteritis 47
thiazide-type diuretics 113
thoracic aortic aneurysm 40, 48
thoracic outlet syndrome 51–52
thoracic symptoms of PAD 40–41
thromboangiitis obliterans 115
thrombophlebitis 49–50
thrombosis 44
thrombus formation leading to
  occlusion 1
tibioperoneal disease, surgical
  management 171–173
tibioperoneal endovascular
  interventions 153–155
ticagrelor 117
tissue perfusion, physiological
  testing 65–66
tobacco use
  cessation and PAD risk 14–15,
    114–116
  risk factor for atherosclerosis 2
  risk factor for PAD 13–15, 38
tocilizumab 101
toe–brachial index 64
tooth loss, PAD risk and 19

transcutaneous oximetry
  ($TcPO_2$) 66
transient ischemic attack (TIA) 38
transient monocular blindness 38

u
ulcers 44, 120
  arterial 49
  characteristics of common leg and
    foot ulcers 49–50
  ischemic 49
  neuropathic 49
  non-healing 3
  venous 49
ultrasonic Doppler
  development of 59
  physiological testing 59–60
ultrasonic duplex scanning 67–69
ultrasound imaging, detection of
  subclinical
  atherosclerosis 1–2
unfractionated heparin
  (UFH) 139–141
uvula, split 46

v
varenicline 115
vascular disease 45
vascular laboratory accreditation 69
vascular laboratory assessment of
  PAD 57–69
  anatomic studies 57
  duplex scanning 67–69
  functional studies 58
  hemodynamic studies 57–58
  physiological testing 58–66
vascular rings in the aortic arch 40
vasculitis 45, 96, 101–102
vasospasm 1
venous ulcers 49
vertebral artery bruits 48
vitamin E supplementation 129
vorapaxar 117

w

Walking Impairment Questionnaire
(WIQ)   42, 43, 119
warfarin   116
wheezing   40

wounds, lower extremity wound
care   120–121

x

xanthelasma   46